# Calc Hero:

## Ultimate Infusion Calculation Mastery

Charles F. Swearingen

# DEDICATION

I would like to dedicate this text to the clinicians at a truly remarkable flight program. One of the first skills I mastered while under their guiding influence was calculating infusions. I was given an equation by a few of the best educators at this flight program, and soon realized it was similar one I had used before. After combining these two equations I found an incredibly useful method for calculating infusion problems, both forwards and backwards.

Without Daniel Turner, Kevin King, Mark Randall, and Jason Rogers, I wouldn't have mastered this skill so quickly and with such precision. Thank you guys, and all of the AirCare team in Jackson, Mississippi with the University of Mississippi Medical Center. I feel that all my medical accomplishments, I owe to the desire for success you all instilled in me: Donna Norris, Todd Perry, Dr. Bob Galli, Bill Bailey, and Paul Boackle. I still work hard to make sure I make you all proud. Thank you for teaching me, from the bottom of my heart.

# CONTENTS

## FIND AN ERROR?

Let us know by filling out the form associated with this QR code. You can also email us at errors@medspx.com.

[Intentionally left Blank]

# Reviewers:

Thank you for your hard work in looking for my errors after I compiled this text. Without you, people would think I'm an idiot. I appreciate your time and effort. Thank you.

**Chris Elliott**
**Critical Care Paramedic and Clinical Educator**
Tupelo, Mississippi
North Mississippi Medical Center

**Walid Al-jabiri, Flight Paramedic**
Jamestown, New York
Fluvanna Fire Department
Mercy Flight of Western New York

**Noel Couch, Flight Paramedic**
Tucson, Arizona
Native Air (An Air Methods Company)

**J. R. Waller, Flight Paramedic**
Waverly, Nebraska
Midwest MedAir

**Susan Hollowell, Flight RN**
Goldsboro, North Carolina
Air Methods

# 1 TRADTIONAL MEDICATION INFUSION CALCULATION

Clinicians are often intimidated by the math that occurs in everyday medical practice. Patient safety depends on the clinician's ability to calculate medications correctly and in a timely manner. It does not matter if you are primarily using a programmable ('smart') intravenous (IV) pump or one that is not programmable-- you have a responsibility to your patients to routinely, and with a high level of accuracy, calculate medication infusions in order to assure patient's safety.

The Traditional Methodologies

There have traditionally been three different methods of calculating medication infusion problems: formula, proportion expressed as a ratio, and proportion expressed as a fraction (dimensional analysis). These each require a solid understanding of algebra, which can cause problems for many clinicians who fail to maintain these skills. I will provide these methods as an option for those who routinely utilize them, and then will present my HYBRID METHOD for calculating medication infusion problems.

## **FORMULA**:

(D/H) x V = Amount of medication to be given

D = desired dose
H = dose on hand
V = Vehicle- tablet or fluid

*Example 1.1: You are ordered to administer Benadryl 50 mg PO. You have 25 mg capsules available.*

D = 50 mg
H = 25
V = Capsule

(D/H) x V = Amount of medication to be given
(50 mg/25 mg) x capsule = 2 capsules

*Example 1.2: You want to administer 10 mcg/kg/min of dopamine to your patient. You have a 250 cc NS bag with 400 mg of dopamine in it. Your patient is 100 kg. How fast will you run this on the IV pump (cc/hr)?*

D = 10 mcg/kg/min
H = 40 mg
V = 250 cc NS

(D/H) x V = Amount to give
([10 mcg][100 kg][60 min/hr]/[400 mg][1000mcg/mg]) x 250 cc NS

= 37.5 cc/hr

This works great for simple tablets, capsules, or PO liquids as in Example 1 above. However, when you need to calculate a medication infusion problem, units can easily be left out- leading to a potential medication error. For instance in Example 1.2, you would have had to know to multiply the dose by the patient's weight in kg, as well as to multiply by 60 since the rate needs to be in cc/hr and the dose was referenced in minutes. Next you would have needed to convert the milligrams of the drug on hand into micrograms. And finally, you would need to multiply by 250 (as in 250 cc of NS) to yield 37.5 cc/hr. There were WAY TOO many assumptions in Example 1.2. If you are skilled at using this method, then by all means keep using it. If this confused the crap out of you, then keep reading. I'll get you on the right track.

## RATIO AND PROPORTION:

H : V :: D : x

**Extremes**

$$H : V :: D : x$$

**Means**

D = desired dose
H = dose on hand
V = Vehicle- tablet or fluid
x = amount to give

Multiply the means and set them equal to the product of the extremes:

Hx = VD, therefore,
x = (VD/H)

(*psst!*- this is the same thing as "(D/H) x V = Amount to give")

So, let's apply this "different" method to the same examples.

### Example 1.1: You are ordered to administer Benadryl 50 mg PO. You have 25 mg capsules available.

D = 50 mg
H = 25
V = Capsule
x = Amount to give

x = (VD/H)
x = (1 capsule x 50 mg)/(25 mg)
x = 2 capsules

*Example 1.2:* **You want to administer 10 mcg/kg/min of dopamine to your patient. You have a 250 cc NS bag with 400 mg of dopamine in it. Your patient is 100 kg. How fast will you run this on the IV pump (cc/hr)?**

D = 10 mcg/kg/min
H = 40 mg
V = 250 cc NS.
x = Amount to give

x = (VD/H)
x = [(250 cc NS)( 10 mcg)(100 kg)(60 min/hr)]/[(400 mg)(1000mcg/mg)]
x = 37.5

Again, how is this not confusing even when you get the numbers in all the right places? Assume you do get the numbers in the right spots, well then you'll need a refresher on mathematical order of operations to crunch the numbers to arrive at the correct calculation. To top it off, to actually obtain the numbers in all the right spots, you'd have to make the same assumptions as before (converting minutes to hours and milligrams to micrograms).

There has to be a better way- and there *is*. Stay with me.

## FRACTIONAL (DIMENSIONAL ANALYSIS):

To practice dimensional analysis, you simply write out the quantities next to one another, add in conversion factors to ensure the quantities are in 'like' systems, and then compute. Let's jump right into the previous two examples. Start with the basic matrix below.

*Example 1.1: You are ordered to administer Benadryl 50 mg PO. You have 25 mg capsules available.*

| 50 mg | 1 capsule | |
|-------|-----------|---|
| | 25 mg | = 2 capsules |

That seems easy enough, but let's try the more difficult question.

*Example 1.2: You want to administer 10 mcg/kg/min of dopamine to your patient. You have a 250 cc NS bag with 400 mg of dopamine in it. Your patient is 100 kg. How fast will you run this on the IV pump (cc/hr)?*

| 10 mcg | 100 kg | 60 min | 250 cc NS | 1 mg |
|--------|--------|--------|-----------|------|
| Kg x min | 1 | 1 hr | 400 mg | 1000 mcg |

| 10 m̶g̶ | 100 k̶g̶ | 60 m̶i̶n̶ | 250 cc | 1 m̶g̶ | |
|--------|--------|--------|--------|-------|---|
| K̶g̶ x m̶i̶n̶ | 1 | 1 hr | 400 m̶g̶ | 1000 m̶c̶g̶ | = 37.5 cc/hr |

So you can see here that this is a much better way to account and manage these problems, but it still requires an good understanding of algebra. These methods are simply not user friendly. In the upcoming chapters, I will assist you in understanding how to identify numbers in a medication calculation problem and then to apply them to a template that will turn this difficult task into an easy one. In not much time at all, you'll be crushing these types of calculation problems.

# 2 THE ANATOMY OF INFUSION CALCULATION PROBLEMS

The field and practice of medicine is riddled with data. Blood pressure, heart rate, respiratory rate, serum pH, as well as many others represent common data encountered daily. Other data is calculated based on simple observations to account for all different kinds of physiological phenomena. This book will focus on the skill of calculating medication infusions and offer a methodology to crush all of your future infusion calculation problems.

Anatomy of Infusion Calculation

Medication infusion problems can be some of the toughest in critical care transport to answer. Often this is because the clinician does not gain a solid foundation in the skill of medication calculation and delivery in their training or it degrades due to insufficient practice. When approaching these problems, it is important to understand the patterns that repeat from problem to problem. In this chapter, we will identify and discuss these repeated patterns which will be referred to as the medication infusion problem's 'anatomy.'

The basic anatomy of an infusion calculation problem is simple and there are three components: DOSE, CONCENTRATION, and RATE. Medication problems will be presented in word problem format and it will be the clinician's job to identify the anatomy so that the appropriate values can be calculated. It is therefore necessary to be able to identify the dose, concentration, and rate in a medication infusion problem.

VOLUME, AMOUNT & TIME

The key to identifying these various "anatomical' components lies in knowing how the quantities volume, amount, and time relate to one another. Each of the three major anatomical components of a medication infusion problem (dose, concentration, and rate) are defined by two of these three quantities.

## **IDENTIFYING CONCENTRATION**:

Concentration is composed of a volume of fluid (250 cc NS bag, or 250 cc D5W glass bottle) with an amount of a medication (in grams, milligrams, micrograms, units, etc) dissolved into it. This is the easiest component to find in a test question because any infusion must start with a medication, right? Well, anytime you take an amount of medication and dump it into a fluid (like in an IV bag), then you have a concentration. Typically, these two quantities (volume and medication amount) are seen adjacent to one another.

The concentration, therefore, is simply the division of the amount of drug into a particular volume of fluid. I like to call the volume portion of the concentration the "fluid vehicle". Concentration will almost ALWAYS be provided in a medication infusion calculation question. Therefore, you will almost ALWAYS have the volume of fluid and an amount of drug will be divided into.

# IDENTIFY MEDICATION INFUSION PROBLEM ANATOMY

1. DOSE = "It's where its AT" as in AT = amount over time
2. CONC = Look for a fluid vehicle with medication in it
3. RATE = volume given over time, cc/hr or gtts/min

Let's Practice!

Read the following test question and answer the questions to follow:

> **2.1** Your adult GI bleed patient has become hypotensive. Following adequate fluid resuscitation, the patient's systolic blood pressure is still less than 80 mmHg. You decide to administer dopamine at 10 mcg/kg/min. The patient weighs 156 pounds. At what rate will you start this infusion if you have 400mg of dopamine in a 250cc bag of normal saline?

1. Can you pick out the concentration (CONC)? HINT: it is an amount of drug in a volume of fluid. Write down the two numbers that together represents concentration in the notes section to the right.
2. What is the desired DOSE?

**Answer and Rationale:**

If you choose 400mg and 250cc of normal saline as the CONC and 10 mcg/kg/min as the DOSE, then you are correct. See how easy it is?! Let's take a look at the other numbers and assign 'anatomical' labels to them.

**BP of 80**: This plays no part in the calculation of the infusion. This is simply the indication for using dopamine. Test writers will throw extra numbers in a problem to confuse and distract you. You're looking for dose numbers, concentration numbers, rate numbers, and known conversion factor numbers (time, volume, weight, or amount conversions) and labeling them.

**10 mcg/kg/min**: This is an amount over time, which is a DOSE. Sure, its mcg per kg, but that is still an amount, it is just weight based, and then goes into the patient each minute. A drug amount over time is always a dose.

**Patient weight of 156 pounds**: So here you would need to convert pounds into kilograms since the dose (10 mcg/kg/min) is weight based (has a "per kilogram" component), but we will talk about the HOW TO later. For now just focus on identifying the anatomical parts.

**400mg Dopamine**: This is the amount of drug added to an infusion bag, therefore is half of the concentration 'anatomy".

**250cc of normal saline**: This is the fluid that the drug will be put into and mixed into the solution that will be administered to the patient. This represents the other half of concentration "anatomy".

Once you understand that these numbers can only be related to dose, rate, concentration, or conversion, then it becomes easy to pick them out of a test question. So as you proceed through this text, continue to label the numbers as either dose, concentration, rate, or common conversion factor.


## IDENTIFYING DOSE:

Dose is composed of an amount of a medication (in grams, milligrams, micrograms, units, etc) over a period of time (per min, or per hour). Finding the dose in a provided medication infusion problem is as simple as remembering where the dose is "AT". The acronym 'AT' stands for amount and time, helping you to remember that dose is quantified by an amount of a drug and time.

It is important to remember that some dosages are weight based and others are not. The problem itself will tell you whether the medication desired is weight based or not. An interesting finding with respect to weight is the fact that DOSE is the only factor of the three anatomical parts that is weight based. This means if you see a 'kg' anywhere in the problem, it is most certainly associated with the DOSE anatomical element.

Again, a dose is typically an amount of drug (mg, mcg, g, etc.) that is delivered to a patient over time (min, hour). Sometimes, as with IV bolus administration, the time can be very short (over a few seconds like in an IV push) or almost instantaneous (like with a rapid IV push, adenosine, for example). Other times, a medication mixture (or concentration) must infuse over longer periods of time such as minutes or hours. This is the bread and butter to infusion calculation problems in that it isn't an instantaneous push, it's a very slow push over time.

Identifying dose is pretty easy because you normally have to have drug dosages memorized, or otherwise can access them from a protocol manual, flip book, or phone app. Even if these dosages are not committed to memory, simply looking for a drug amount set over time will help you label a particular dose number in a test question.

Let's Practice Again!

Yes, we will do this a lot in this text so have a pencil or pen handy so you can participate and take notes as you learn.

Read the following test question and answer the questions to follow:

**Example 2.2** You have a patient experiencing an acute myocardial infarction. The patient weighs approximately 72 kg. The patient is to be placed on a nitroglycerin drip. The glass bottle of nitroglycerin has 250cc of D5W in it. The patient is to receive 6mcg/min, and there is exactly 50mg in the glass bottle of nitroglycerin. How fast will you run this infusion?

1. Can you pick out the dose?   HINT: it is an amount of drug given over a particular time period.
2. What is the CONC?

**Answer and Rationale:**

If you chose 6 mcg/min as the dose and 50 mg in 250 cc NS as the concentration, then you are exactly correct. 6 mcg/min is the only option that is an amount of a drug over a time period, and therefore is the dose. 50 mg in 250 cc NS is the concentration since it represents a medication being dissolved into a fluid vehicle.

## IDENTIFYING RATE:

Rate is the function relating a volume of fluid (with medicine in it) with time (per min, or per hour, etc). In easy, right-to-left medication infusion problems, rate is typically what you are looking to calculate. If you have a desired dose in mind, and you know how you will mix it, then all you need is to calculate and identify the rate that achieves that does with that concentration. When you are given a medication infusion problem, look for a volume over time (such as cc/hr or gtts/min) to clue you into finding the rate

The only thing that makes finding these components difficult is that there are several little things that go together making a complex system. However, if you first UNDERSTAND the components, and second PRACTICE identifying them, then you're on your way to perfection of medical infusion calculation.

Rate is easy to find because it is simply a volume (cc, mL, or gtts) of fluid that is administered over time (min or hr). Therefore, in an exam question we would look for cc/hr. This is a common rate used by in– hospital clinicians and critical care transport clinicians. In the ambulance, you may see the gtts/hr because they are using gravity, not a pump. Some progressive EMS services have IV pumps and those practitioners will be more familiar with cc/hr.

Please note, sometimes rate will not be included if an exam question is asking for rate. Said differently, an exam writer cannot give you a rate in the problem if they are going to ask you to calculate rate for the answer.

Let's Practice!

Read the following test question and answer the questions to follow:

---

**Example 2.3** You arrive at a local ER to transport an ICU patient to a larger ICU. The patient has norepinephrine infusing at 22 cc/hr and she is 159kg. You note that the norepinephrine IV bag is a 500cc bag of normal saline with 2 mg of norepinephrine inside. What rate is the patient receiving?

---

1. What is the RATE?
2. What is the concentration?

**Answer and Rationale:**

Did you choose 22 cc/hr as the rate? Then you are correct! Did you choose 2 mg of norepi in a 500 cc bag of NS as the concentration? Then, again, you are correct! See?, this stuff isn't so hard. These are simple identifiers that ultimately compose a complex system– and that is what is difficult. However, as long as you know these smaller components, you can more easily tackle the calculation.

**Review Time**

Please fill in the below table by returning to problems 2.1, 2.2, and 2.3 and filling in their various components into the blank table.

|      | Dose | Conc | Rate |
|------|------|------|------|
| **2.1** |      |      |      |
| **2.2** |      |      |      |
| **2.3** |      |      |      |

# 3 DIRECTIONAL FLOW

Let's be practical for just a moment. When are you ever going to need to work a medication dosing or infusion problem? Just take a second to think when you'll really need to do this. There are two primary instances where you may need to exercise this skill:

1. You need to mix a medication and deliver it to the patient.
2. You are picking up a patient that already has an infusion running and you want to ensure that the patient is receiving the correct dosage.

If you think about it directionally, you have two options: forward and backward. This is an important concept to understand because later I will offer a method that can be used to calculate any medical infusion calculation problem successfully based on the direction of "flow".

Let's take a look at this.

**(DOSE) (CONC) = (RATE)**

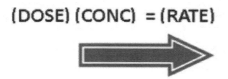

When you are attempting to find the RATE, you must already have the dose and concentration. The dose is easily obtained either from a flip book, a protocol manual, a textbook, or from memory. Once you arrive at the desired dose, then you need to choose the appropriate intravenous fluid. Typically normal saline or lactated ringers are common isotonic crystalloids used to mix medication infusions. To deliver medicines intravenously you must mix the medication in some fluid vehicle.

Once a medication is injected into an IV bag, it immediately develops a property called concentration. Concentration is a quantity characterized by a specific volume of fluid and a specific amount of medication. If you change the amount of medication in the bag, by adding more medication, you would in effect be increasing the concentration. If you were instead to add more fluid to the IV bag, then you would be weaken, or lessening, the concentration.

Once you have identified the dose you wish to administer (desired dose) as well as define the amount of medication that will be injected into a fluid vehicle (concentration), you are ready to deliver the medication. A simple calculation is all that stands between you and successful completion of a medication infusion problem. I call problems like these, where you are looking to calculate rate from a given dose and concentration, "Forward Direction" medication calculation problems.

### Now Reverse!

The next direction would be the "Backwards Direction", or the direction you would want to use if you needed to calculate whether a patient was receiving the correct dose of an infusion already started. As you would expect, it looks like this:

# (DOSE) (CONC) = (RATE)

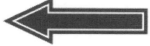

The big picture is to understand what you are trying to solve for and typically it's one of two things: rate or dose. You solve for *rate* when you are going to start a new infusion, and you solve for *dose* when you are checking to see that the infusion someone else has already begun is correct. If it isn't correct, then you'll have to make the adjustment on the IV pump.

Concentration will NEVER be what you are looking for, at least not in the practical clinical world, nor on most exams. Sure, perhaps you'll see one on a test during your career, where they are asking you to calculate the concentration, but it is not necessary in practice. Typically you will want to know rate and the problem will give you concentration and dose, or you will want the dose and the problem will give you concentration and rate.

These are the two most common question archetypes:

1. Use CONC and DOSE to get RATE (Forward)
2. Use CONC and RATE to get DOSE (Backward)

## Let's Practice!

Let's consider the GI patient chapter 2 (example 2.1), only this time you are picking them up to transport them to a bigger hospital.

Read the following test question and answer the questions to follow:

**Question 3.1** You are picking up an adult trauma patient who has become hypotensive from a spinal injury. The patient is receiving 60 mcg/min of Neosynepherine and is running at 40cc/hr on the IV pump. The patient weighs 102 kg. You look at the IV bag and note that there are 10mg of Neosynepherine in 250cc of normal saline. Is the patient receiving the correct dose?

1. What is the direction of this problem?
2. Can you pick out the concentration?
3. Can you pick out the rate?

**Answer and Rationale:**

If you answered 20cc/hr for rate and 400mg/250cc for concentration, then you have got the intuitive flow concept down. In this case, you'll need to use concentration and rate to calculate the actual dose the patient is receiving, and compare it to what the hospital says the patient is receiving. So, you see, we have to calculate the correct dose and make sure it matches what the hospital is reporting, and if it's wrong, then we need to change the IV pump to the correct rate.

# 4 THE HYBRID METHOD

The hybrid method represents a strategy rather than a formula. A formula is rigid and inflexible, whereas this Hybrid Method (HM) allows for flexibility in approaching medication infusion problems. The flexibility comes in the form of two terms in the template that may be included or excluded depending the dosing of the medication. For instance, some medications are administered in 'unit per kilo per hour' while others are 'unit per kilo per minute.' Still others are administered 'unit per hour' as well as a few other options. This method quickly and easily allows the clinician to include or exclude two different terms making it flexible for ANY medication infusion calculation.

I would like to introduce the Hybrid Method for calculating medication infusion problems.

$$\frac{(DD)(KG)(60)(VOL)}{(DRUG)} = \text{cc/hr or gtts/min}$$

You'll see on the top of the divisor line, 'DD' which stands for the desired dose that has been ordered by the MD, DO, PA, or nurse practitioner; is in your protocols; or otherwise is identified in a test question.

Next is the term, 'KG', which stands for kilogram. You include this term in any medication being administered based on weight. If the medication is not weight based, then the 'KG' term would be eliminated from the template.

The third term is '60' and is included in the template if the medication being administered is based on minutes. If the medication being administered is a 'per hour' the '60' would be eliminated from the template.

The last term on the top of the divisor line is 'VOL' and represents the volume of the ??fluid vehicle the medication is injected into.

The last term on the left side of the equals sign is the 'DRUG' term. It represents the amount of medication that is injected into the fluid vehicle. Trivially, VOL and DRUG together represent the concentration. You should note that the 'KG' and the '60' terms are the terms which are flexible because their presence will vary from medication to medication.

When the template is simplified, or computed, the result is an infusion rate expressed in BOTH cc/hr or gtts/min. This is where this method derives its namesake. It hybridizes two different equations: one that arrives at cc/hr and one that arrives at gtts/min. There is a caveat. For the gtts/min version to be true, the clinician has to be using a 60 drop set. See, the '60' term in the template represents 60 minutes in an hour (specific to the cc/hr version) and 60 drops in one cc (specific to the gtts/min version). It's like two people with the same first name, they are called the same thing, but they are completely different people. The value of the result, no matter which version you use, will always be the same. It is hybridized. Please see the two following sets of examples to prove the hybridization concept.

**Example 4.1:** You are to administer 20 micrograms per kilogram per minute of dopamine to a hypotensive patient. The drug is mixed in standard concentration with 400 mg in 250 cc normal saline. The patient weighs 100 kg. At what rate will you run this infusion?

Step 1: Write out the blank template.

Step 2: Identify anatomy and assign values to the template. Note the "60" has the units cc/hr.

$$\frac{[20 \text{ mcg}]}{[\text{kg} \times \text{min}]} \left|[100 \text{ kg}]\right| \frac{[60 \text{ min}]}{[1 \text{ hr}]} \left|\frac{[250 \text{ cc}]}{[400 \text{ mg}]}\right| = \text{cc/hr}$$

Step 3: Synchronize the dose and concentration by adding 3 zeros if the units do not match.

$$\frac{[20 \text{ mcg}]}{[\text{kg} \times \text{min}]} \left|[100 \text{ kg}]\right| \frac{[60 \text{ min}]}{[1 \text{ hr}]} \left|\frac{[250 \text{ cc}]}{[400\,000 \text{ mcg}]}\right| = \text{cc/hr}$$

Step 4: Cross out like terms.

$$\frac{[20 \text{ mcg}]}{[\text{kg} \times \text{min}]} \left|[100 \text{ kg}]\right| \frac{[60 \text{ min}]}{[1 \text{ hr}]} \left|\frac{[250 \text{ cc}]}{[400\,000 \text{ mcg}]}\right| = \text{cc/hr}$$

Step 5: Compute.

$$\frac{[20 \text{ mcg}]}{[\text{kg} \times \text{min}]} \left|[100 \text{ kg}]\right| \frac{[60 \text{ min}]}{[1 \text{ hr}]} \left|\frac{[250 \text{ cc}]}{[400\,000 \text{ mcg}]}\right| = 75 \text{ cc/hr}$$

**Example 4.2:** You are to administer 20 micrograms per kilogram per minute to a hypotensive patient. The drug is mixed in standard concentration with 400 mg in 250 cc normal saline. The patient weighs 100 kg. Use a 60 gtts set for gravity flow administration. At what rate will you run this infusion? Note this is the same problem as Example 1.

Step 1: Write out the blank template.

Step 2: Identify anatomy and assign values to the template. Note the "60" has the units gtts/cc.

$$\frac{[20 \text{ mcg}]}{[\text{kg} \times \text{min}]} \Bigg| \frac{[100 \text{ kg}]}{} \Bigg| \frac{[60 \text{ gtts}]}{[1 \text{ cc}]} \Bigg| \frac{[250 \text{ cc}]}{[400 \text{ mg}]} = \text{gtts/min}$$

Step 3: Synchronize the dose and concentration by adding 3 zeros if the units do not match.

$$\frac{[20 \text{ mcg}]}{[\text{kg} \times \text{min}]} \Bigg| \frac{[100 \text{ kg}]}{} \Bigg| \frac{[60 \text{ gtts}]}{[1 \text{ cc}]} \Bigg| \frac{[250 \text{ cc}]}{[400\,000 \text{ mcg}]} = \text{gtts/min}$$

Step 4: Cross out like terms.

$$\frac{[20 \text{ mcg}]}{[\text{kg} \times \text{min}]} \Bigg| \frac{[100 \text{ kg}]}{} \Bigg| \frac{[60 \text{ gtts}]}{[1 \text{ cc}]} \Bigg| \frac{[250 \text{ cc}]}{[400\,000 \text{ mcg}]} = \text{gtts/min}$$

Step 5: Compute.

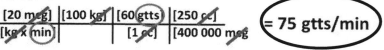

$$\frac{[20 \text{ mcg}]}{[\text{kg} \times \text{min}]} \Bigg| \frac{[100 \text{ kg}]}{} \Bigg| \frac{[60 \text{ gtts}]}{[1 \text{ cc}]} \Bigg| \frac{[250 \text{ cc}]}{[400\,000 \text{ mcg}]} = 75 \text{ gtts/min}$$

As you can see, the 60 min/hr term and the 60 gtts/min term both arrive at the same computed value: 75. This is the beauty of the Hybrid Method- it allows for two different approaches to be merged, or hybridized, into one with the simple caveat that to use the "gtts/min" version, you need to be using a 60 drop gravity set. A 60 drop gravity set simply means that it takes 60 drops (or gtts) to make a single cc (or mL).

## Special Rules of the Hybrid Method

Once you trust that these two equations hybridize to yield the exact same values, then it is time to further discuss the unique rules, of the Hybrid Method. Recall the 'KG' term can be included into the template (if the medication is weight based) or excluded (if it is not a weight based medication). The beauty of every test question you'll ever face is that it has to tell you whether it's weight based or not. If the question doesn't mention that the medication is weight based, then you can routinely and safely assume it is not. In the practical world, you'll need to know offhand whether the medicine is weight based. You may memorize all of your medication doses, keep a cheat sheet, use a flip book, or rely on an app to have this information available to you.

The second caveat has to do with the 60 term. The only time you leave the 60 term in the template is when the dosing calls for the medication to be delivered "per minute." If it is a "per hour" medication dose, the 60 term is excluded from the template.

The third and final caveat has to do with the relative magnitude of the dosing units and the concentration units. If you are dosing a medication in micrograms, chances are you injected an amount of that medication that is in milligrams (1000 times that of the dose). For instance, consider that dopamine is dosed in 20 mcg/kg/min, or micrograms. Recall that dopamine's standard concentration is 400 milligrams in 250 cc. The difference in micrograms (dose) and milligrams (concentration) is 1000x. By simply identifying the magnitude of dose and concentration, you can tell easily if they are the same magnitude or if they are separated by 1000x. One way to think of this is to question if the units 'match' or not. If the units of dosing magnitude and concentration magnitude match, then do nothing. If the units of dosing magnitude are different (smaller) than the concentration magnitude (bigger) then simply add 3 zeroes to the concentration value (as if to multiply it by 1000). This synchronizes the dosing and concentration magnitudes. After this step, the template is ready to be simplified, calculated.

Recall from the examples 1 and 2 (which?) the problem:

Step 1: Write out the blank template.

Step 2: Identify anatomy and assign values to the template. Note the "60" has the units gtts/cc.

$$\frac{[20 \text{ mcg}]}{[\text{kg} \times \text{min}]} \bigg| \frac{[100 \text{ kg}]}{} \bigg| \frac{[60 \text{ gtts}]}{[1 \text{ cc}]} \bigg| \frac{[250 \text{ cc}]}{[400 \text{ mg}]} = \text{gtts/min}$$

Step 3: Synchronize the dose and concentration by adding 3 zeros if the units do not match.

$$\frac{[20 \text{ mcg}]}{[\text{kg} \times \text{min}]} \bigg| \frac{[100 \text{ kg}]}{} \bigg| \frac{[60 \text{ gtts}]}{[1 \text{ cc}]} \bigg| \frac{[250 \text{ cc}]}{[400\,000 \text{ mcg}]} = \text{gtts/min}$$

As you can see in step 2, the DD is 20 micrograms (mcg) but the DRUG available is in milligrams (400 mg). When this is the case, the clinician must be sure to synchronize the units of the DD and the available DRUG by simply adding 3 zeros to the end of the DRUG value (or multiply by 1000x). Doing so essentially equalizes the units.

Hybridization of these two equations that results in the same <u>absolute value</u> for both cc/hr and gtts/min. This makes for an easy transition from those using gravity sets (from perhaps an ambulance transport) to a setting that uses IV pumps (like an ER or ICU). It makes the math seamless by simply using a template to organize the various numerical elements of a medical infusion problem.

We have discussed the anatomy of a medical infusion calculation problem and introduced the Hybrid Method as a way to place 'anatomical' values into a template. Now it's time to marry the skills of identifying medical infusion question anatomy with the ability to assign the these anatomical values to a term in the template. It will be important to use the three whatevers....., or rules, rules when applying anatomy to the template. After this has been accomplished, we simply crunch the numbers.

# 7 steps to achieve the infusion rate using the template

1. Always, write out the template first.

2. Identify Anatomy

   a. Identify the desired dose from the test question or real world problem; then write this value (no units) over the DD of the template.

   b. If the medication to be administered is weight based, then write the patient's weight in kilograms over the KG term. If it is not weight based, place an 'X' over the KG term in the template and do not use it in the template calculation.

   c. If the medication to be administered 'per min' then put a check mark over the 60 term to indicate it should be used in the calculation. If it is a 'per hour' drug, place an 'X' over the 60 term in the template and do not use it in the template calculation.

   d. Identify the medication concentration by identifying an amount of medication (DRUG term) injected into a fluid amount (typically an IV bag or large syringe). Assign the fluid volume (plus the fluid volume used to inject the medication into the IV bag or syringe) to the VOL term. Assign the amount of injected medication to the DRUG term.

3. Identify if the dose and concentration drug magnitudes match. If they are both the same magnitude, then do nothing. If the dose is 1000 times smaller than the concentration magnitude, then add 3 zeros to the DRUG term as to multiply it by 1000, which makes the two magnitudes equal.

4. Finally, compute.

## Let's Practice!

Let's re-consider the GI patient chapter 2.

**Examples 2.1/4.3**   Your adult GI bleed patient has become hypotensive. Following adequate fluid resuscitation, the patient's blood pressure is still low (less than 80). You decide to administer dopamine at 10 mcg/kg/min. The patient weighs  156 lbs. What rate will you start this infusion if you have 400mg of dopamine in a 250cc bag of normal saline?

Step 1: Write out the blank template.

$$\frac{(DD) \mid (KG) \mid (60) \mid (VOL)}{\qquad\qquad\qquad\quad (DRUG)} = cc/hr$$

Step 2: Identify anatomy and assign values to the template.
Keep the '60' term for "per min" drugs and keep the KG if it is weight based.

$$\frac{\overset{10}{(DD)} \mid \overset{71}{(KG)} \mid (60) \mid \overset{250}{(VOL)}}{\qquad\qquad\qquad\quad \underset{400}{(DRUG)}} = xxxx \; cc/hr$$

Step 3: Synchronize the dose and concentration by adding
3 zeros if the units do not match.

$$\frac{\overset{10}{(DD)} \mid \overset{71}{(KG)} \mid (60) \mid \overset{250}{(VOL)}}{\qquad\qquad\qquad\quad \underset{400\;000}{(DRUG)}} = xxxx \; cc/hr$$

Step 4: COMPUTE.

$$\frac{\overset{10}{(DD)} \mid \overset{71}{(KG)} \mid (60) \mid \overset{250}{(VOL)}}{\qquad\qquad\qquad\quad \underset{400\;000}{(DRUG)}} = \boxed{75 \; cc/hr}$$

Let's consider the AMI patient chapter 2.

**Examples 2.2/4.4** You have a patient experiencing an acute myocardial infarction. The patient weighs approximately 72 kg. The patient is to be placed on a nitroglycerin drip. The glass bottle of nitroglycerin has 250cc of D5W in it. The patient is to receive 6mcg/min, and there is exactly 50mg in the glass bottle of nitroglycerin. How fast will you run this infusion?

Step 1: Write out the blank template.

$$\frac{(DD) \mid (KG) \mid (60) \mid (VOL)}{\mid \mid (DRUG)} = cc/hr$$

Step 2: Identify anatomy and assign values to the template.
Keep the '60' term for "per min" drugs and keep the KG if it is weight based.

$$\frac{\overset{6}{(DD)} \mid \overset{}{(\cancel{KG})} \mid (60) \mid \overset{250}{(VOL)}}{\mid \mid \underset{50}{(DRUG)}} = xxxx \; cc/hr$$

Step 3: Synchronize the dose and concentration by adding 3 zeros if the units do not match.

$$\frac{\overset{6}{(DD)} \mid \overset{}{(\cancel{KG})} \mid (60) \mid \overset{250}{(VOL)}}{\mid \mid \underset{50 \;\; 000}{(DRUG)}} = xxxx \; cc/hr$$

Step 4: COMPUTE.

$$\frac{\overset{6}{(DD)} \mid \overset{}{(\cancel{KG})} \mid (60) \mid \overset{250}{(VOL)}}{\mid \mid \underset{50 \;\; 000}{(DRUG)}} = \boxed{1.8 \; cc/hr}$$

**Let's Do two more!**

---

**Example 4.5** A neuro patient is to be administered Propofol for continued sedation. The patient weighs approximately 110 kg. The glass bottle of Propofol has 100cc with 1000 mg Propofol in it. The patient is to receive 12 mcg/kg/min. How fast will you run this infusion?

---

Step 1: Write out the blank template.

$$\frac{(DD) \mid (KG) \mid (60) \mid (VOL)}{\qquad\qquad\qquad (DRUG)} = cc/hr$$

$$\frac{\overset{12}{(DD)} \mid \overset{110}{(KG)} \mid (60) \mid \overset{100}{(VOL)}}{\qquad\qquad\qquad \underset{1000}{(DRUG)}} = xxxx \; cc/hr$$

Step 3: Synchronize the dose and concentration by adding 3 zeros if the units do not match.

$$\frac{\overset{12}{(DD)} \mid \overset{110}{(KG)} \mid (60) \mid \overset{100}{(VOL)}}{\qquad\qquad\qquad (DRUG)} = xxxx \; cc/hr$$

1000 **000**

Step 4: COMPUTE.

$$\frac{\overset{12}{(DD)} \mid \overset{110}{(KG)} \mid (60) \mid \overset{100}{(VOL)}}{\qquad\qquad\qquad (DRUG)} = \boxed{7.9 \; cc/hr}$$

1000 **000**

**Example 4.6** Your trauma patient is receiving a Versed drip for continued sedation. The patient weighs approximately 88 kg. You currently have two 5 mg vials of versed that you have injected into a 250 cc bag of NS. The patient is to receive 4 mg/hr. How fast will you run this infusion?

Step 1: Fill in the template.

NOTE: DRUG is 10 (not 5 mg) because there are two 5mg vials we added to the 250 cc of NS. The dose calls for mg/hr, therefore, the '60' and 'KG' terms are NOT included in the calculation

$$\frac{(DD) \mid (KG) \mid (60) \mid (VOL)}{\mid \mid (DRUG)} = cc/hr$$

Step 2: Identify anatomy and assign values to the template.
Keep the '60' term for "per min" drugs and keep the KG if it is weight based.

$$\frac{4 \quad\quad 250}{(DD) \mid \cancel{(KG)} \mid \cancel{(60)} \mid (VOL)} = xxxx \ \mathbf{cc/hr}$$
$$\frac{}{\mid \mid (DRUG)}$$
$$10$$

Step 3: Synchronize the dose and concentration by adding 3 zeros if the units do not match.

$$\frac{4 \quad\quad 250}{(DD) \mid \cancel{(KG)} \mid \cancel{(60)} \mid (VOL)} = xxxx \ \mathbf{cc/hr}$$
$$\frac{}{\mid \mid (DRUG)}$$
$$10 \quad \mathbf{No\ zeros\ added}$$

Step 4: COMPUTE.

$$\frac{4 \quad\quad 250}{(DD) \mid \cancel{(KG)} \mid \cancel{(60)} \mid (VOL)} = \boxed{\mathbf{100\ cc/hr}}$$
$$\frac{}{\mid \mid (DRUG)}$$
$$10 \quad \mathbf{No\ zeros\ added}$$

# 5 RETROCACLULATION

There are many times as a clinician you will be assuming care of patients from another clinician. In these times, it's your responsibility to ensure that any medications that are infusing are being administered at the appropriate dose, which is associated with a specific rate. Traditionally, these are the most difficult medication infusion problems because they require you to calculate backwards, or retrocalculate. The Hybrid Method's template sets up an easy platform to identify the question 'anatomy', assign them to the appropriate terms, and compute.

There are two directions that were previously mentioned: forward direction problems and backward direction problems. The forward direction is designed to calculate an infusion rate. These are situations where the test question provides you with the ordered dose, the weight (if necessary), and the concentration. Alternatively, in the real world, you would know the dose (from memory or looking it up in a resource) and you'd mix the medication in a fluid vehicle, thus you'd know the concentration.

This chapter will focus on the second direction, or the backwards direction. Consider the situation where you arrive to transport a patient receiving a vasopressor. The dose is reported to be 20 mcg/kg/min of dopamine. You transport the patient to the receiving facility and the MD taking over care asks why you were only giving 2 mcg/kg/min. It is our responsibility to ENSURE what is reported is actually being delivered. Never assume the report is correct and always double check.

To be able to ensure a medication is infusing at the correct rate and dose, it is important you retrocalculate the infusing medication and compare the actual dose. Obviously, they should closely match. With the Hybrid Method retrocalculation is very easy. Once practiced 10-20 times, we are seeing students being able to perform the retrocalculation using only a calculator and their memory.

Retrocalculation can be summarized by the phrase, "multiply, then divide, divide, divide." This describes (1) multiplying the rate by the amount of drug in the IV bag or syringe (DRUG), then (2) dividing by the volume of concentration (VOL), then (3) dividing by 60 (if a 'per min' drug) and finally (4) dividing by KG (if it's weight based). This calculation results in the desired dose the patient is actually receiving.

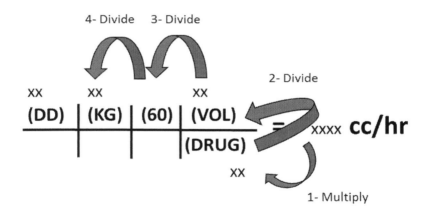

The trick here is to KNOW the dosing units- either from the report, memory, or some resource. This helps you synchronize the terms in the template. For instance, consider a patient you receive from a sending facility where dopamine is infusing. You receive a report stating the dosing is 20 mcg/kg/min. From this, it is evident that it's weight based, administered 'per min', and the dosing units are in micrograms. The only other piece of information you need is to look at the IV bag or syringe and note if the injected medication matches the dosing units. If the medication units in the bag do not match the dose units (mg in bag and dose is in micrograms), then you need to add 3 zeros to the DRUG value.

Let me prove this works. Re-consider the situation mentioned earlier where the MD discovered you were only giving 2 mcg/kg/min of dopamine instead of 20 mcg/kg/min. Reportedly, the sending facility was administering 20 mcg/kg/min. Once you observe the IV pump, you notice the rate is 20 mcg/kg/min. You consider maybe they got the rate and dose backwards (yes- this actually happens more often than you think). The patient is 100 kg In this case, I will provide representations of the IV bag, IV pump, and drug dosages. So, let's set this up step by step.

STEP 1: Write out the template.

$$\frac{(DD) \mid (KG) \mid (60) \mid (VOL)}{\mid \quad \mid \quad \mid (DRUG)} = cc/hr$$

STEP 2: Obtain the current infusion rate and place it in the template.

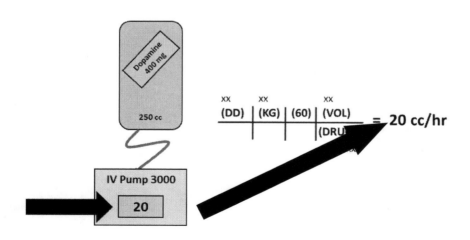

## STEP 3: Obtain DRUG (make sure corners match)

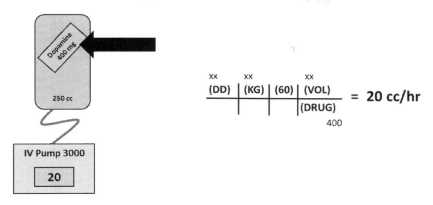

## STEP 4: Match the corners

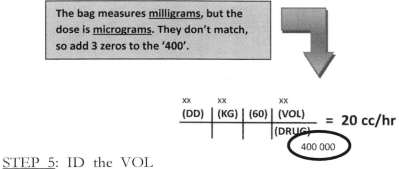

The bag measures **milligrams**, but the dose is **micrograms**. They don't match, so add 3 zeros to the '400'.

## STEP 5: ID the VOL and write on template

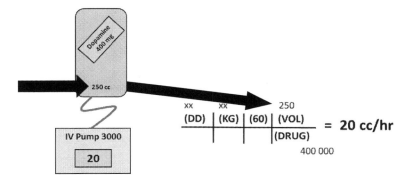

STEP 6: Add 60 if it's a 'per min' drug

> The dose was in mcg/kg/min, therefore the 60 participates in the calculation.

$$\frac{\begin{array}{c|c|c|c} xx & xx & \checkmark & 250 \\ (DD) & (KG) & (60) & (VOL) \\ & & & (DRUG) \end{array}}{400\,000} = 20\ cc/hr$$

STEP 7: Add KG if the dose is weight based

> The dose was in mcg/kg/min, therefore patient's weight must participate.

$$\frac{\begin{array}{c|c|c|c} xx & 100 & \checkmark & 250 \\ (DD) & (KG) & (60) & (VOL) \\ & & & (DRUG) \end{array}}{400\,000} = 20\ cc/hr$$

STEP 8: Calculate by "multiply, then divide, divide, divide"

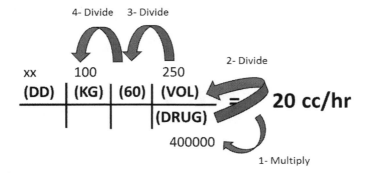

34

The Solution:

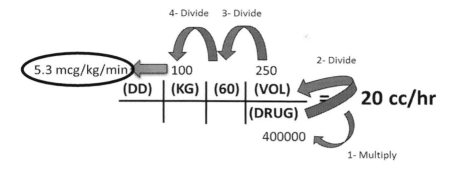

As you can see, the patient was actually receiving 5.3 mcg/kg/min instead of "20 mcg/kg/min" that was reported. Entry into your calculator should look as follows:

- [20] x [400000][Equals]
- [divided by][250] [Equals]
- [divided by][60] [Equals]
- [divided by][100] [Equals]

The result is 5.3 mcg/kg/min. This means the sending facility was under-dosing the patient by a magnitude of 4x, and was failing to trigger the vasopressor effect of dopamine. Later, we will discuss how to troubleshoot inconsistencies, but first let's review and practice.


## SUMMARY:

### Retrocalculation Steps

1. Write out the template.
2. Obtain the current infusion rate from the IV pump and write this value over the cc/hr term.
3. Obtain the amount of drug from the IV bag or syringe (on a syringe pump) and write this amount under the DRUG term.
4. Consider units of the dose amount and the concentration

amount. If they do not match, add 3 zeros to the DRUG term- as if it was multiplied by 1000 which accounts for the difference in magnitude.

5. Obtain the fluid volume the medication was injected into (plus the fluid volume used to actually inject the medication) and write this value over the VOL term.

6. If the medication to be administered is 'per min' then put a check mark over the 60 term to indicate it should be used in the calculation. If it is a 'per hour' drug, place an 'X' over the 60 term in the template and do not use it in the template calculation.

7. If the medication to be administered is weight based, then write the patient's weight in kilograms over the KG term. If it is not weight based, place an 'X' over the KG term in the template and do not use it in the template calculation.

8. Calculate by multiplying RATE and DRUG, then hit equal, then divide that result by VOL, then divide that result by 60 (if a 'per minute' drug), and finally divide that result by the patient's weight (if the medication is weight based).

**5.1** You are transporting an AMI patient on nitroglycerin. The patient weighs approximately 90 kg. The IV pump reads 20 cc/hr, and the IV bottle has 250 of D5W with 50 mg of nitro in it. You recall that nitro is administered in mcg/min. What is the dose that the patient is currently receiving?

Step 1: Write out the blank template.

$$\frac{(DD) \mid (KG) \mid (60) \mid (VOL)}{\mid \mid (DRUG)} = cc/hr$$

Step 2: Identify anatomy and assign values to the template.
Keep the '60' term for "per min" drugs and keep the KG if it is weight based.

$$\frac{X \qquad\qquad \checkmark\ 250}{(DD) \mid (K\!G) \mid (60) \mid (VOL)} = 20\ cc/hr$$
$$(DRUG)\ 50$$

Step 3: Synchronize the dose and concentration by adding 3 zeros if the units do not match.

$$\frac{X \qquad\qquad \checkmark\ 250}{(DD) \mid (K\!G) \mid (60) \mid (VOL)} = 20\ cc/hr$$
$$(DRUG)$$
$$50\ \mathbf{000}$$

Step 4: COMPUTE (Multiply, then Divide, Divide, ~~Divide~~).

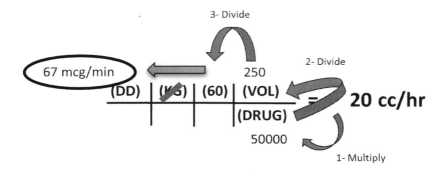

37

**5.2** As you arrive to transport a 50 y/o in hypertensive crisis, you note labetalol infusion running a 2 cc/hr. The sending facility reports the infusion is administering 2 mg/min of labetalol. The patient's weight is 220 lbs. The infusion bag has 1 gram of labetalol in a 500 cc. What dose is the patient receiving?

Step 1: Write out the blank template.

$$\frac{(DD) \mid (KG) \mid (60) \mid (VOL)}{\mid \mid (DRUG)} = cc/hr$$

Step 2: Identify anatomy and assign values to the template.
Keep the '60' term for "per min" drugs and keep the KG if it is weight based.

$$\frac{\overset{X}{(DD)} \mid \overset{\cancel{}}{(\cancel{KG})} \mid \overset{\checkmark}{(60)} \mid \overset{500}{(VOL)}}{\mid \mid \underset{1}{(DRUG)}} = 2 \ cc/hr$$

Step 3: Synchronize the dose and concentration by adding
3 zeros if the units do not match.

$$\frac{\overset{X}{(DD)} \mid \overset{\cancel{}}{(\cancel{KG})} \mid \overset{\checkmark}{(60)} \mid \overset{500}{(VOL)}}{\mid \mid \underset{1 \ \mathbf{000}}{(DRUG)}} = 2cc/hr$$

Step 4: COMPUTE (Multiply, then Divide, Divide, ~~Divide~~).

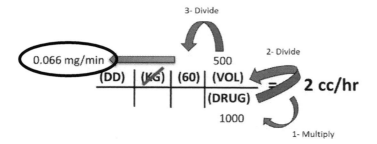

They are nowhere near the correct dose. At this concentration, 60 cc/hr is needed to deliver 2 mg/min.

**5.3** You are transporting a patient with atrial fib who is currently receiving an infusion of diltiazem. The IV pump is currently at 10 cc/hr and the medical staff reports the patient is receiving a dose of 10 mg/hr. The patient weighs 73 kg. You look up at the infusion bag and note there is 250 cc NS with 300 mg of diltiazem in it. What dosage of diltiazem is the patient currently receiving?

Step 1: Write out the blank template.

$$\frac{(DD) \mid (KG) \mid (60) \mid (VOL)}{\mid \mid (DRUG)} = cc/hr$$

Step 2: Identify anatomy and assign values to the template.
Keep the '60' term for "per min" drugs and keep the KG if it is weight based.

$$\frac{X \qquad\qquad 250}{(DD) \mid (\cancel{KG}) \mid (\cancel{60}) \mid (VOL)}{\mid \mid (DRUG) \atop 300} = 10 \ cc/hr$$

Step 3: Synchronize the dose and concentration by adding 3 zeros if the units do not match.

$$\frac{X \qquad\qquad 250}{(DD) \mid (\cancel{KG}) \mid (\cancel{60}) \mid (VOL)}{\mid \mid (DRUG)} = 10 \ cc/hr$$

300  **No zeros needed- corners match**

Step 4: COMPUTE (Multiply, then Divide, Divide, ~~Divide~~).

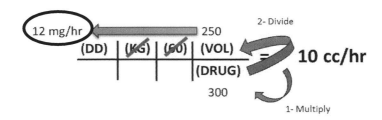

They are slightly incorrect on their dosage. They are actually administering 12 mg/hr, not 10. This may not need adjusting, but be sure to inform the receiving facility of the correct dose.

# 6 ADVANCED TOPICS

In this chapter, we will discuss several advanced topics. These will include Quick Draw calculations, on-the-fly adjustments, infusions involving units (instead of grams, milligrams, or micrograms), and finally we will explore percent solutions. In my experience, these topics are not well understood, and I wanted to take the time to explain them and how to troubleshoot these topics.

## QUICK DRAW CALCULATIONS

The method I have provided allows the clinician to move forwards and backwards in calculating rate and dose, respectively. That makes this method incredibly powerful and useful. This text contains 100 shift practice sessions, each with 3 medication infusion practice problems. To transcend good to great and even beyond expert, it takes practice. Luckily, we are seeing expert-like skill after practicing 30-50 practice problems successfully. This is why this text delivers the primary content, then offers 50 full-explanation practice problems, and then begins a year's worth of shift practice sessions. We want you to have ample, exemplary, challenging, and consistent practice at this skill. Within a few days, you'll be great at this, and by the year's end, you'll be an expert.

To be able to quickly calculate medication infusion problems, you'll need to practice to the point where you can see the main equation in your head:

$$\frac{(DD)(KG)(60)(VOL)}{(DRUG)} = cc/hr$$

Once you can see it in your head, you'll be able to search your surroundings and resources for all the elements you need to start typing into your calculator. Memorizing the doses and units of common IV infusion medications you either come in contact to or otherwise initiate, can provide you with quick access (recall) to dosing information. Practicing the use of the flexibility of the KG and the 60 terms in the Hybrid Method base equation. Simply observing the amount of a medication in an IV bag gives you the concentration. Identifying the current IV pump rate starts the backwards directional question. By harnessing these simple resources, Quick Draw calculations can happen much faster than you anticipate.

Forward Quick Draw

To utilize the forward flow and derive the rate at which you want to deliver a particular medication at a particular concentration, again, you will have to memorize the dosages and dose units of common medications administered via continuous infusion. See the list below (for a useful list of common medications administered via continuous infusion) and the QR code to the right (for a link to a flashcard data set that I created for you) to practice recalling this critical information.

MCG/KG/MIN:
- Dopamine 2-20 mcg/kg/min
- Dobutamine 2-20 mcg/kg/min
- Propofol 5-50+ mcg/kg/min
- Nitroprusside 0.3-10 mcg/kg/min

MCG/MIN:

- Epinephrine 2-10 mcg/min
- Nitroglycerin 10-100+ mcg/min
- Norepinepherine 1-30 mcg/min
- Neosynepherine 50-200 mcg/min

MG/MIN:

- Labetalol 2-10 mg/min
- Lidocaine 1-4 mg/min50-200

MG/HR:

- Diltiazem 10-15 mg/hr
- Cardene 5-15 mg/hr

Remember, the dose units will give insight to the need to include the KG and/or the 60 term in the Hybrid Method. Dose units including mcg/kg/min indicates the need for both terms. Problems with the dose units mcg/min and mg/min only need the 60 term. The problem with the dose units mg/hr does not need either of the flexible terms in the Hybrid Method.

During the peer review of this text, it was mentioned that some medications, such as neosynepherine or Isuprel, can be administered in mcg/kg/min and mcg/min, depending on which source you read. Recall the problem has to deliver this information to you. In this text if this information is not provided, then use the above dose units as a standard. In the real world, use what you are familiar with: if you know the dose range of Isuprel using mcg/min, then use it. If you are familiar with the dose range for Isuprel using mcg/kg/min, then use that one. If ever the case you have a 'per kg', then you simply add in the KG term in the hybrid equation. The method is no different.

Once you have the dose, KG term, and 60 term identified and situated, you then need to identify the concentration elements in the problem or in your medical kit. The concentration elements are the easiest to find in my opinion, and once you have these identified, you have all you need to start calculating. Let's see how this looks.

**6.1: Consider a patient needing a nitroglycerin infusion of 10 mcg/min. You see the bottle in the picture to the right. The following is the <u>thought</u> and <u>action</u> process needed to calculate the correct rate in under 20 seconds (literally I just did it to get a time).**

| | |
|---|---|
| THINK: | What is the dose for nitro: 10-100 mcg/min. |
| ACTION: | Type [10] in calculator, then hit [x]. |
| THINK: | Is this weight based? No, it isn't. |
| ACTION: | Move on to the 60 term. |
| THINK: | Is this a "per min" drug? Yes, it is. |
| ACTION: | Type [60] into the calculator and then hit [=] then [x]. |
| THINK: | How much fluid was initially in the fluid vehicle? In this case, there is 250 in the nitro bottle. |
| ACTION: | Type [250] into the calculator and then hit [=] then [divide by]. |
| THINK: | How much medication is in the fluid vehicle? In this case, 50 mg are in the nitro bottle. Also think here if the corners match, and here they don't so add 3 zeros to the medication value. |
| ACTION: | Type [50, 000] into the calculator and then hit [=]. |

---

**ANSWER: 3 cc/hr**

---

The result (3 cc/hr) is the rate needed to achieve the dose of 10 mcg/min with the concentration of 50 mg in 250 cc.

To utilize the backward flow and derive the actual DOSE the patient is receiving, you'll need to look to the IV pump for the rate and the IV bag for the concentration elements. In actuality, this can be done faster than the forward direction. It is still important to have memorized common drug dosages, so be sure to do that.

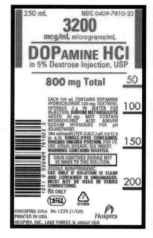

**6.2: Consider another patient that is receiving 40 cc/hr of dopamine. Look to the label to the right for other pertinent information. The patient weights 70 kg. Here is how the thought and action process should go to make this a quick and easy calculation.**

| | |
|---|---|
| THINK: | What is the current IV pump rate: 40 cc/hr |
| ACTION: | Type [40] in calculator, then hit [x]. |
| THINK: | How much medication is in the fluid vehicle? In this case, 800 mg are in the IV bag. Also- think if the corners match, and here they don't so add 3 zeros to the medication value (800,**000**). |
| ACTION: | Type [800000] into the calculator and then hit [=] then [divided by]. |
| THINK: | How much fluid was initially in the fluid vehicle? In this case, there is 250 in the IV bag. |
| ACTION: | Type [250] into the calculator and then hit [=] then [divide by]. |
| THINK: | Is this a "per min" drug? Yes, it is. |
| ACTION: | Type [60] into the calculator and then hit [=] then [divide by]. |
| THINK: | Is this weight based? Yes, the patient weighs 70 kg. |
| ACTION: | Type [70] into the calculator and then hit [=]. |

---

**ANSWER: 30.4 cc/hr**

The result (30.4 mcg/kg/min) is the dose the patient is actually receiving. This is a pediatric dosage of dopamine. Do not let weird concentrations throw you off. Train yourself to simply look at the number, pick out anatomy, plug into the template, match the corners, and then calculate.

## ON-THE-FLY ADJUSTMENTS

Once you successfully calculate a medication infusion problem, you're left with powerful tools at both ends of the template. Following successful calculation, and assuming you do not add more medication or fluid to the IV bag (or change the concentration), the dose and rate take on an interval relationship. This means the distance between the two are always equal. Let me show you what I mean.

Earlier in the book we had the solution below. We started with an IV pump rate (10 cc/hr). We then retrocalculated to arrive at a dose of 12 mg/hr being delivered. The math here is correct for this diltiazem infusion.

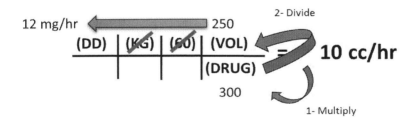

The ends of the template hold powerful tools: they tell us that for every change of 10 cc/hr on the pump will increase the dosage by another 12 mg/hr. So, if we increased the IV pump to 20 cc/hr, we could expect a new dosage of 24 mg/hr. If we increased the IV pump to 30 cc/hr, we could expect a new dosage of 36 mg/hr.

This interval relationship arms us with a powerful weapon: the ability to make on-the-fly changes with pinpoint accuracy. It highlights even further the importance of setting up the problem correctly- which is the role of the Hybrid Method template. Then, by harnessing the power of the interval relationship between dose and rate, quick changes can be made with very little effort exerted.

Let's practice a few.

**6.3 A patient is receiving a dose of 5 mcg/min from a rate of 15 cc/hr. The patient should be receiving a dose of 15 mcg/min. What adjustment could you make to arrive at the correct dose for this patient?**

Answer:

The interval here is between dos and rate- 5 mcg/min : rate of 15 cc/hr. If the patient should be receiving 15 mcg/min and they are only receiving 5 mcg/min, then they are only receiving a third of the dose. To correct, multiply the rate by 3 to arrive at 45 cc/hr. This rate would deliver a dose of 15 mcg/min.

**6.4 A patient is receiving a dose of 2 mg/min from a rate of 7 cc/hr. The patient should be receiving a dose of 1 mg/min. What adjustment could you make to arrive at the correct dose for this patient?**

Answer:

The interval here is between dos and rate- 2 mg/min : rate of 7 cc/hr. If the patient should be receiving 1 mg/min and they are receiving 2 mg/min, then they are receiving twice the dose. To correct, reduce the rate by half to arrive at 3.5 cc/hr. This rate would deliver a dose of 1 mg/min.


You see, on-the-fly adjustments can come in very handy in the patients already receiving a continuous infusion where the dosage is not accurate. By simply understanding the interval relationship between dose and rate in a successfully calculated medication infusion problem, you can harness the ability to make quick changes to the IV pump and zero in on the actual desired dose.

# 7 INITIAL PRACTICE

Once you have reviewed and studied the material enough, then you'll want to start on your journey towards becoming a Calc Hero right here. In the following pages, you will be exposed to 34 different medication infusion problems. Each one will be broken down and shown how to be successfully worked. Pearls and insights will be added where appropriate to truly nail down teaching points.

This chapter is designed around a medication infusion problem. Work it however you wish, but we will explain it in terms of the Hybrid Method. Once you complete this initial practice, ideally over a time span of 2-10 days, then begin the shift practice sessions in chapter 8.

> **7.1** You are to infuse Tridil. The protocol calls for 15 mcg/min. 50 mg has been injected into a 500 cc D5W IV bag. The patient weighs 100 kg. To ensure this dose, what rate should the IV pump be programmed to?

Step 1: Write out the blank template.

$$\frac{(DD) \mid (KG) \mid (60) \mid (VOL)}{\mid \mid (DRUG)} = cc/hr$$

Step 2: Identify anatomy and assign values to the template.
Keep the '60' term for "per min" drugs and keep the KG if it is weight based.

$$\frac{\overset{15}{(DD)} \mid \cancel{(KG)} \mid (60) \mid \overset{500}{(VOL)}}{\mid \mid \underset{50}{(DRUG)}} = xxxx \ cc/hr$$

Step 3: Synchronize the dose and concentration by adding 3 zeros if the units do not match.

$$\frac{\overset{15}{(DD)} \mid \cancel{(KG)} \mid (60) \mid \overset{500}{(VOL)}}{\mid \mid (DRUG)} = xxxx \ cc/hr$$
$$50 \ \mathbf{000}$$

Step 4: COMPUTE.

$$\frac{\overset{15}{(DD)} \mid \cancel{(KG)} \mid (60) \mid \overset{500}{(VOL)}}{\mid \mid (DRUG)} = \boxed{9 \ cc/hr}$$
$$50 \ \mathbf{000}$$

Step 1: Write out the blank template.

$$\frac{(DD) \mid (KG) \mid (60) \mid (VOL)}{\mid \mid (DRUG)} = cc/hr$$

Step 2: Identify anatomy and assign values to the template.
Keep the '60' term for "per min" drugs and keep the KG if it is weight based.

$$\frac{5 \qquad\qquad 250}{(DD) \mid (\cancel{KG}) \mid (\cancel{60}) \mid (VOL)} = xxxx \; cc/hr$$
$$\frac{}{\mid \mid (DRUG)}$$
$$20$$

Step 3: Synchronize the dose and concentration by adding
3 zeros if the units do not match.

$$\frac{5 \qquad\qquad 250}{(DD) \mid (\cancel{KG}) \mid (\cancel{60}) \mid (VOL)} = xxxx \; cc/hr$$
$$\frac{}{\mid \mid (DRUG)}$$
$$20 \quad \textbf{No zeros added}$$

Step 4: COMPUTE.

$$\frac{5 \qquad\qquad 250}{(DD) \mid (\cancel{KG}) \mid (\cancel{60}) \mid (VOL)} = \boxed{25 \; cc/hr}$$
$$\frac{}{\mid \mid (DRUG)}$$
$$20 \quad \textbf{No zeros added}$$

**7.3** Your hypotensive patient is currently receiving norepinephrine at a rate of xxx with 5 mg mixed into a 100 cc NS IV bag. The patient is 150 lbs. What dose is the patient currently receiving?

Step 1: Write out the blank template.

$$\frac{(DD) \mid (KG) \mid (60) \mid (VOL)}{\mid \mid (DRUG)} = cc/hr$$

Step 2: Identify anatomy and assign values to the template.
Keep the '60' term for "per min" drugs and keep the KG if it is weight based.

$$\frac{X \qquad \checkmark \quad 100}{(DD) \mid (\cancel{KG}) \mid (60) \mid (VOL)} = 6 \ cc/hr$$
$$\frac{}{\mid \mid (DRUG)}$$
$$5$$

Step 3: Synchronize the dose and concentration by adding
3 zeros if the units do not match.

$$\frac{X \qquad \checkmark \quad 100}{(DD) \mid (\cancel{KG}) \mid (60) \mid (VOL)} = 6 \ cc/hr$$
$$\frac{}{\mid \mid (DRUG)}$$
$$5 \ 000$$

Step 4: COMPUTE (Multiply, then Divide, Divide, ~~Divide~~).

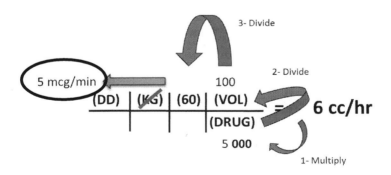

Step 1: Write out the blank template.

$$\frac{(DD) \mid (KG) \mid (60) \mid (VOL)}{\mid \mid (DRUG)} = cc/hr$$

Step 2: Identify anatomy and assign values to the template.
Keep the '60' term for "per min" drugs and keep the KG if it is weight based.

$$\frac{\overset{2}{(DD)} \mid \overset{95}{(KG)} \mid (60) \mid \overset{250}{(VOL)}}{\mid \mid \underset{50}{(DRUG)}} = xxxx \ \mathbf{cc/hr}$$

Step 3: Synchronize the dose and concentration by adding 3 zeros if the units do not match.

$$\frac{\overset{2}{(DD)} \mid \overset{95}{(KG)} \mid (60) \mid \overset{250}{(VOL)}}{\mid \mid (DRUG)} = xxxx \ \mathbf{cc/hr}$$

50 **000**

Step 4: COMPUTE.

$$\frac{\overset{2}{(DD)} \mid \overset{95}{(KG)} \mid (60) \mid \overset{250}{(VOL)}}{\mid \mid (DRUG)} = \boxed{57 \ cc/hr}$$

50 **000**

**7.5** A patient is in shock and you need to administer epinephrine. You will administer 2 mcg/ min. Your plan is to mix 1 mg of 1:1000 epi into a 250 cc IV bag. The patient is 58 kg. What rate will you run this infusion at?

Step 1: Write out the blank template.

$$\frac{(DD) \mid (KG) \mid (60) \mid (VOL)}{\mid \mid (DRUG)} = cc/hr$$

Step 2: Identify anatomy and assign values to the template.
Keep the '60' term for "per min" drugs and keep the KG if it is weight based.

$$\frac{2 \quad \quad \quad 250}{(DD) \mid (K\cancel{G}) \mid (60) \mid (VOL)}{\mid \mid (DRUG)} = xxxx \ cc/hr$$
$$1$$

Step 3: Synchronize the dose and concentration by adding 3 zeros if the units do not match.

$$\frac{2 \quad \quad \quad 250}{(DD) \mid (K\cancel{G}) \mid (60) \mid (VOL)}{\mid \mid (DRUG)} = xxxx \ cc/hr$$
$$1 \quad 000$$

Step 4: COMPUTE.

$$\frac{2 \quad \quad \quad 250}{(DD) \mid (K\cancel{G}) \mid (60) \mid (VOL)}{\mid \mid (DRUG)} = \boxed{30 \ cc/hr}$$
$$1 \quad 000$$

**7.6** You are transporting a patient currently receiving dobutamine at a rate of 25 cc/hr. The 500 cc IV bag has a label that reads " 350 mg of dobutamine". The patient weight is 121 kg. What dose is the patient receiving?

Step 1: Write out the blank template.

$$\frac{(DD) \mid (KG) \mid (60) \mid (VOL)}{\mid \mid (DRUG)} = cc/hr$$

Step 2: Identify anatomy and assign values to the template.
Keep the '60' term for "per min" drugs and keep the KG if it is weight based.

$$\frac{X \quad\; 121 \quad\checkmark\quad 500}{(DD) \mid (KG) \mid (60) \mid (VOL) \atop \mid \mid (DRUG) \atop 350} = 25 \;\; cc/hr$$

Step 3: Synchronize the dose and concentration by adding
          3 zeros if the units do not match.

$$\frac{X \quad\; 121 \quad\checkmark\quad 500}{(DD) \mid (KG) \mid (60) \mid (VOL) \atop \mid \mid (DRUG)} = 25 \; cc/hr$$

350 **000**

Step 4: COMPUTE (Multiply, then Divide, Divide, Divide).

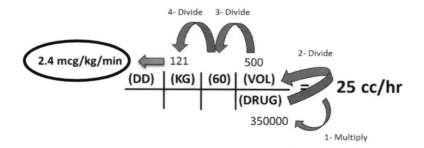

**7.7** A neuro patient is in your care and propofol is chosen for continued sedation. You decide to start with 10 mcg/kg/min. The bottle comes with 1000 mg in 100 cc. The patient weighs 85 kg. What rate will you run this infusion at?

Step 1: Write out the blank template.

$$\frac{(DD) \mid (KG) \mid (60) \mid (VOL)}{\mid \quad \mid \quad \mid (DRUG)} = cc/hr$$

Step 2: Identify anatomy and assign values to the template.
Keep the '60' term for "per min" drugs and keep the KG if it is weight based.

$$\frac{\overset{10}{(DD)} \mid \overset{85}{(KG)} \mid (60) \mid \overset{100}{(VOL)}}{\mid \quad \mid \quad \mid \underset{1000}{(DRUG)}} = xxxx \ cc/hr$$

Step 3: Synchronize the dose and concentration by adding
3 zeros if the units do not match.

$$\frac{\overset{10}{(DD)} \mid \overset{85}{(KG)} \mid (60) \mid \overset{100}{(VOL)}}{\mid \quad \mid \quad \mid (DRUG)} = xxxx \ cc/hr$$

1000 **000**

Step 4: COMPUTE.

$$\frac{\overset{10}{(DD)} \mid \overset{85}{(KG)} \mid (60) \mid \overset{100}{(VOL)}}{\mid \quad \mid \quad \mid (DRUG)} = \boxed{5.1 \ cc/hr}$$

1000 **000**

> **7.8** Labetalol has been chosen for your hypertensive emergency patient. You have 1 gram available and will use a 250 cc IV bag. Your patient weighs 100 kg. You decide to begin the dose at 3 mg/min. What rate will you run this infusion at?

Step 1: Write out the blank template.

$$\frac{(DD) \mid (KG) \mid (60) \mid (VOL)}{\mid \quad \mid \quad \mid (DRUG)} = cc/hr$$

Step 2: Identify anatomy and assign values to the template.
Keep the '60' term for "per min" drugs and keep the KG if it is weight based.

$$\frac{\overset{3}{(DD)} \mid \cancel{(KG)} \mid (60) \mid \overset{250}{(VOL)}}{\mid \quad \mid \quad \mid \underset{1}{(DRUG)}} = \text{xxxx } \mathbf{cc/hr}$$

Step 3: Synchronize the dose and concentration by adding
3 zeros if the units do not match.

$$\frac{\overset{3}{(DD)} \mid \cancel{(KG)} \mid (60) \mid \overset{250}{(VOL)}}{\mid \quad \mid \quad \mid \underset{1 \quad 000}{(DRUG)}} = \text{xxxx } \mathbf{cc/hr}$$

Step 4: COMPUTE.

$$\frac{\overset{3}{(DD)} \mid \cancel{(KG)} \mid (60) \mid \overset{250}{(VOL)}}{\mid \quad \mid \quad \mid \underset{1 \quad 000}{(DRUG)}} = \boxed{\textbf{45 cc/hr}}$$

**7.9** The IV pump reads "30 cc/hr". Your patient is receiving a continuous infusion of neosynepherine. You have injected 10 mg into a 250 cc NS IV bag. The patient is 65 kg. What dose is the patient receiving?

Step 1: Write out the blank template.

$$\frac{(DD) \mid (KG) \mid (60) \mid (VOL)}{\mid \mid (DRUG)} = cc/hr$$

Step 2: Identify anatomy and assign values to the template.
Keep the '60' term for "per min" drugs and keep the KG if it is weight based.

$$\frac{X \qquad\qquad \checkmark \quad 250}{(DD) \mid (\cancel{KG}) \mid (60) \mid (VOL)}{\mid \mid (DRUG)} = 30 \text{ cc/hr}$$
10

Step 3: Synchronize the dose and concentration by adding
3 zeros if the units do not match.

$$\frac{X \qquad\qquad \checkmark \quad 250}{(DD) \mid (\cancel{KG}) \mid (60) \mid (VOL)}{\mid \mid (DRUG)} = 30 \text{ cc/hr}$$
10 **000**

Step 4: COMPUTE (Multiply, then Divide, Divide, ~~Divide~~).

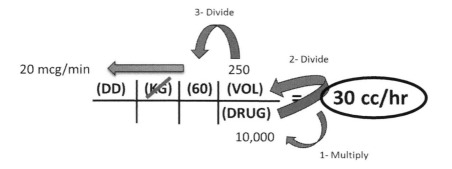

3- Divide

2- Divide

20 mcg/min

$$\frac{(DD) \mid (\cancel{KG}) \mid (60) \mid (VOL)}{\mid \mid (DRUG)} = \boxed{30 \text{ cc/hr}}$$
250
10,000

1- Multiply

**7.10** Heparin 20,000 units in 500 mL D5W is ordered to run at 1,000 units/hour. The patient is 104 kg. What rate will you run this infusion at?

Step 1: Write out the blank template.

$$\frac{(DD) \mid (KG) \mid (60) \mid (VOL)}{\mid \quad \mid \quad \mid (DRUG)} = cc/hr$$

Step 2: Identify anatomy and assign values to the template.
Keep the '60' term for "per min" drugs and keep the KG if it is weight based.

$$\frac{\overset{1000}{(DD)} \mid \overset{}{(\cancel{KG})} \mid (\cancel{60}) \mid \overset{500}{(VOL)}}{\mid \quad \mid \quad \mid \underset{20,000}{(DRUG)}} = \text{xxxx } cc/hr$$

Step 3: Synchronize the dose and concentration by adding 3 zeros if the units do not match.

$$\frac{\overset{1000}{(DD)} \mid (\cancel{KG}) \mid (\cancel{60}) \mid \overset{500}{(VOL)}}{\mid \quad \mid \quad \mid (DRUG)} = \text{xxxx } cc/hr$$

20,000   **No zeros added**

Step 4: COMPUTE.

$$\frac{\overset{1000}{(DD)} \mid (\cancel{KG}) \mid (\cancel{60}) \mid \overset{500}{(VOL)}}{\mid \quad \mid \quad \mid (DRUG)} = \boxed{25 \ cc/hr}$$

20,000   **No zeros added**

**7.11** A MD wants you to continue a fentanyl drip for an intubated cancer patient targeting 300 mcg/hr. Five (5) mg of fentanyl was injected into a 500 cc D5W IV bag. The patient weighs 58 kg. What rate will you run this infusion at?

Step 1: Write out the blank template.

$$\frac{(DD) \mid (KG) \mid (60) \mid (VOL)}{\mid \quad \mid (DRUG)} = cc/hr$$

Step 2: Identify anatomy and assign values to the template.
Keep the '60' term for "per min" drugs and keep the KG if it is weight based.

$$\frac{\overset{300}{(DD)} \mid \cancel{(KG)} \mid \cancel{(60)} \mid \overset{500}{(VOL)}}{\mid \quad \mid \underset{5}{(DRUG)}} = xxxx \; cc/hr$$

Step 3: Synchronize the dose and concentration by adding
3 zeros if the units do not match.

$$\frac{\overset{300}{(DD)} \mid \cancel{(KG)} \mid \cancel{(60)} \mid \overset{500}{(VOL)}}{\mid \quad \mid (DRUG)} = xxxx \; cc/hr$$
5 000

Step 4: COMPUTE.

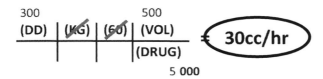

$$\frac{\overset{300}{(DD)} \mid \cancel{(KG)} \mid \cancel{(60)} \mid \overset{500}{(VOL)}}{\mid \quad \mid (DRUG)} = \boxed{30cc/hr}$$
5 000

Step 1: Write out the blank template.

$$\frac{\text{(DD)} \mid \text{(KG)} \mid \text{(60)} \mid \text{(VOL)}}{\mid \mid \text{(DRUG)}} = \text{cc/hr}$$

Step 2: Identify anatomy and assign values to the template.
Keep the '60' term for "per min" drugs and keep the KG if it is weight based.

$$\frac{\text{X} \qquad\qquad \checkmark \quad 250}{\text{(DD)} \mid \text{(K̶G̶)} \mid \text{(60)} \mid \text{(VOL)}}{\mid \mid \text{(DRUG)}_3} = \textbf{13 cc/hr}$$

Step 3: Synchronize the dose and concentration by adding 3 zeros if the units do not match.

$$\frac{\text{X} \qquad\qquad \checkmark \quad 250}{\text{(DD)} \mid \text{(K̶G̶)} \mid \text{(60)} \mid \text{(VOL)}}{\mid \mid \text{(DRUG)}} = \textbf{13 cc/hr}$$
$$\text{3} \quad \textbf{000}$$

Step 4: COMPUTE (Multiply, then Divide, Divide, ~~Divide~~).

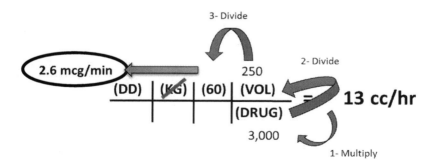

**7.13** A patient is receiving a lidocaine drip. The order is for 3 mg per minute. One gram of lidocaine has been added to a 500 mL IV bag. The patient weighs 110 kg. What rate will you run this infusion at?

Step 1: Write out the blank template.

$$\frac{(DD)\ |\ (KG)\ |\ (60)\ |\ (VOL)}{|\ \ \ \ \ |(DRUG)} = cc/hr$$

Step 2: Identify anatomy and assign values to the template.
Keep the '60' term for "per min" drugs and keep the KG if it is weight based.

$$\frac{\overset{3}{(DD)}\ |\ \cancel{(KG)}\ |\ (60)\ |\ \overset{500}{(VOL)}}{|\ \ \ \ \ |\underset{1}{(DRUG)}} = xxxx\ \textbf{cc/hr}$$

Step 3: Synchronize the dose and concentration by adding 3 zeros if the units do not match.

$$\frac{\overset{3}{(DD)}\ |\ \cancel{(KG)}\ |\ (60)\ |\ \overset{500}{(VOL)}}{|\ \ \ \ \ |\underset{1\ 000}{(DRUG)}} = xxxx\ \textbf{cc/hr}$$

Step 4: COMPUTE.

$$\frac{\overset{3}{(DD)}\ |\ \cancel{(KG)}\ |\ (60)\ |\ \overset{500}{(VOL)}}{|\ \ \ \ \ |\underset{1\ 000}{(DRUG)}} = \boxed{1.5\ \textbf{cc/hr}}$$

**7.14** You need to administer insulin to your DKA patient and decide 3 u/hr is needed. The patient weighs 118 kg. Pharmacy has prepared for you an IV bag of 250 NS with 100 units injected into it. What rate will you run this infusion at?

Step 1: Write out the blank template.

$$\frac{\text{(DD)} \mid \text{(KG)} \mid \text{(60)} \mid \text{(VOL)}}{\mid \mid \text{(DRUG)}} = \text{cc/hr}$$

Step 2: Identify anatomy and assign values to the template.
Keep the '60' term for "per min" drugs and keep the KG if it is weight based.

$$\frac{3 \quad\quad\quad\quad 250}{\text{(DD)} \mid \cancel{\text{(KG)}} \mid \cancel{\text{(60)}} \mid \text{(VOL)}}{\mid \mid \text{(DRUG)} \atop 100} = \text{xxxx cc/hr}$$

Step 3: Synchronize the dose and concentration by adding
3 zeros if the units do not match.

$$\frac{3 \quad\quad\quad\quad 250}{\text{(DD)} \mid \cancel{\text{(KG)}} \mid \cancel{\text{(60)}} \mid \text{(VOL)}}{\mid \mid \text{(DRUG)}} = \text{xxxx cc/hr}$$

100     **No zeros needed**

Step 4: COMPUTE.

$$\frac{3 \quad\quad\quad\quad 250}{\text{(DD)} \mid \cancel{\text{(KG)}} \mid \cancel{\text{(60)}} \mid \text{(VOL)}}{\mid \mid \text{(DRUG)}} = \boxed{7.5 \text{ cc/hr}}$$

100     **No zeros needed**

> **7.15** Nipride is being delivered at 50 cc/hr. The patient weighs 60 kg. On hand, you have 50 mg of Nipride in a 250 cc glass bottle of 0.9% saline. What dose is the patient receiving?

Step 1: Write out the blank template.

$$\frac{\text{(DD)} \;|\; \text{(KG)} \;|\; \text{(60)} \;|\; \text{(VOL)}}{\text{(DRUG)}} = \text{cc/hr}$$

Step 2: Identify anatomy and assign values to the template.
Keep the '60' term for "per min" drugs and keep the KG if it is weight based.

$$\frac{\overset{X}{\text{(DD)}} \;|\; \overset{60}{\text{(KG)}} \;|\; \overset{\checkmark}{\text{(60)}} \;|\; \overset{250}{\text{(VOL)}}}{\underset{50}{\text{(DRUG)}}} = \text{50 cc/hr}$$

Step 3: Synchronize the dose and concentration by adding 3 zeros if the units do not match.

$$\frac{\overset{X}{\text{(DD)}} \;|\; \overset{60}{\text{(KG)}} \;|\; \overset{\checkmark}{\text{(60)}} \;|\; \overset{250}{\text{(VOL)}}}{\underset{50\ \textbf{000}}{\text{(DRUG)}}} = \text{50 cc/hr}$$

Step 4: COMPUTE (Multiply, then Divide, Divide, Divide).

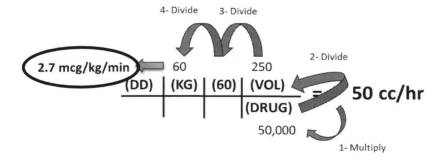

Step 1: Write out the blank template.

$$\frac{(DD)\;|\;(KG)\;|\;(60)\;|\;(VOL)}{|\quad|\quad|(DRUG)} = cc/hr$$

Step 2: Identify anatomy and assign values to the template.
Keep the '60' term for "per min" drugs and keep the KG if it is weight based.

$$\frac{\overset{20}{(DD)}\;|\;\overset{500}{(\cancel{KG})}\;|\;(60)\;|\;(VOL)}{|\quad|\quad|\underset{6}{(DRUG)}} = xxxx\; cc/hr$$

Step 3: Synchronize the dose and concentration by adding 3 zeros if the units do not match.

$$\frac{\overset{20}{(DD)}\;|\;\overset{500}{(\cancel{KG})}\;|\;(60)\;|\;(VOL)}{|\quad|\quad|\underset{6\;000}{(DRUG)}} = xxxx\; cc/hr$$

Step 4: COMPUTE.

$$\frac{\overset{20}{(DD)}\;|\;\overset{500}{(\cancel{KG})}\;|\;(60)\;|\;(VOL)}{|\quad|\quad|\underset{6\;000}{(DRUG)}} = \boxed{50\; cc/hr}$$

**7.17** A patient with a pulmonary embolus is receiving streptokinase. The protocol states 750k IU should be injected into a 200 cc bag of NS and be delivered at 100k IU/hr. Your patient weighs 106 kg. What rate will you run this infusion at?

Step 1: Write out the blank template.

$$\frac{(DD) \mid (KG) \mid (60) \mid (VOL)}{\mid \qquad \mid \qquad \mid (DRUG)} = cc/hr$$

Step 2: Identify anatomy and assign values to the template.
Keep the '60' term for "per min" drugs and keep the KG if it is weight based.

$$\frac{\overset{100}{(DD)} \mid \overset{}{(\cancel{KG})} \mid \overset{200}{(\cancel{60})} \mid (VOL)}{\mid \qquad \mid \qquad \mid \underset{750}{(DRUG)}} = xxxx \; cc/hr$$

Step 3: Synchronize the dose and concentration by adding
3 zeros if the units do not match.

$$\frac{\overset{100}{(DD)} \mid (\cancel{KG}) \mid (\cancel{60}) \mid \overset{200}{(VOL)}}{\mid \qquad \mid \qquad \mid (DRUG)} = xxxx \; cc/hr$$

750    **No zeros needed**

Step 4: COMPUTE.

$$\frac{\overset{100}{(DD)} \mid (\cancel{KG}) \mid (\cancel{60}) \mid \overset{200}{(VOL)}}{\mid \qquad \mid \qquad \mid (DRUG)} = \boxed{26.6 \; cc/hr}$$

750    **No zeros needed**

**7.18** Dopamine is being infused to a hypotensive patient at 15 cc/hr. The patient is 75 kg. Pharmacy has mixed the 500 cc NS IV bag with 1000 mg. What dose is the patient receiving?

Step 1: Write out the blank template.

$$\frac{(DD)\ |\ (KG)\ |\ (60)\ |\ (VOL)}{|\quad|\quad|(DRUG)} = cc/hr$$

Step 2: Identify anatomy and assign values to the template.
Keep the '60' term for "per min" drugs and keep the KG if it is weight based.

$$\frac{\overset{X}{(DD)}\ |\ \overset{75}{(KG)}\ |\ (60)\ |\ \overset{\checkmark\ 500}{(VOL)}}{|\quad|\quad|\underset{1000}{(DRUG)}} = 15\ cc/hr$$

Step 3: Synchronize the dose and concentration by adding 3 zeros if the units do not match.

$$\frac{\overset{X}{(DD)}\ |\ \overset{75}{(KG)}\ |\ (60)\ |\ \overset{\checkmark\ 500}{(VOL)}}{|\quad|\quad|(DRUG)}$$
$$1000\ \mathbf{000} = 15\ cc/hr$$

Step 4: COMPUTE (Multiply, then Divide, Divide, Divide).

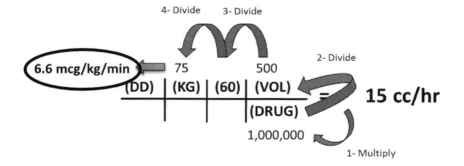

66

**7.19** A patient requires Brevibloc for tachycardia. The order calls for 50 mcg/kg/min. On hand, you have 1500 mg in 500 cc of D5W. The patient weighs 77 kg. What rate will you run this infusion at?

Step 1: Write out the blank template.

$$\frac{(DD) \mid (KG) \mid (60) \mid (VOL)}{\mid \quad \mid \quad \mid (DRUG)} = cc/hr$$

Step 2: Identify anatomy and assign values to the template.
Keep the '60' term for "per min" drugs and keep the KG if it is weight based.

$$\frac{\overset{50}{(DD)} \mid \overset{77}{(KG)} \mid (60) \mid \overset{500}{(VOL)}}{\mid \quad \mid \quad \mid \underset{1500}{(DRUG)}} = xxxx \; cc/hr$$

Step 3: Synchronize the dose and concentration by adding
          3 zeros if the units do not match.

$$\frac{\overset{50}{(DD)} \mid \overset{77}{(KG)} \mid (60) \mid \overset{500}{(VOL)}}{\mid \quad \mid \quad \mid (DRUG)} = xxxx \; cc/hr$$
$$1500\,\mathbf{000}$$

Step 4: COMPUTE.

$$\frac{\overset{50}{(DD)} \mid \overset{77}{(KG)} \mid (60) \mid \overset{500}{(VOL)}}{\mid \quad \mid \quad \mid (DRUG)} = \boxed{77 \; cc/hr}$$
$$1500\,\mathbf{000}$$

**7.20** Amiodarone is infusing for a patient with SVT at 17 cc/hr. The sending facility has provided you with a 500 cc D5W containing 900 mg of amiodarone. The patient weighs 96 kg. What dose is the patient receiving? [recall that Amiodarone dose is in mg/min]

Step 1: Write out the blank template.

$$\frac{(DD) \mid (KG) \mid (60) \mid (VOL)}{\mid \quad \mid \quad \mid (DRUG)} = cc/hr$$

Step 2: Identify anatomy and assign values to the template.
Keep the '60' term for "per min" drugs and keep the KG if it is weight based.

$$\frac{(DD) \mid (K\!\!\!/G) \mid (60) \mid (VOL)\,500}{\mid \quad \mid \quad \mid (DRUG)\,900} = 17 \text{ cc/hr}$$

Step 3: Synchronize the dose and concentration by adding 3 zeros if the units do not match.

$$\frac{(DD) \mid (K\!\!\!/G) \mid (6\!\!\!/0) \mid (VOL)\,500}{\mid \quad \mid \quad \mid (DRUG)\,900} = 17 \text{ cc/hr}$$

No zeros needed: mg = mg

Step 4: COMPUTE (Multiply, then Divide, Divide, ~~Divide~~).

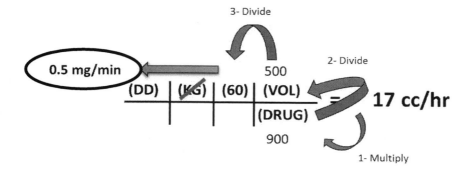

0.5 mg/min

3- Divide

2- Divide

1- Multiply

**7.21** Your patient requires sedation while on the mechanical ventilator, and you decide to administer propofol. On hand, you have a glass bottle with 1000 mg dissolved into a 100 cc lipid emulsion. You decide to start the infusion at 12 mcg/mg/hr. The patient is 80 kg. What rate will you run this infusion at?

Step 1: Write out the blank template.

$$\frac{(DD) \mid (KG) \mid (60) \mid (VOL)}{\mid \mid (DRUG)} = cc/hr$$

Step 2: Identify anatomy and assign values to the template.
Keep the '60' term for "per min" drugs and keep the KG if it is weight based.

$$\frac{\overset{12}{(DD)} \mid \overset{80}{(KG)} \mid (60) \mid \overset{100}{(VOL)}}{\mid \mid \underset{1000}{(DRUG)}} = xxxx \; cc/hr$$

Step 3: Synchronize the dose and concentration by adding
3 zeros if the units do not match.

$$\frac{\overset{12}{(DD)} \mid \overset{80}{(KG)} \mid (60) \mid \overset{100}{(VOL)}}{\mid \mid \underset{1000\,\mathbf{000}}{(DRUG)}} = xxxx \; cc/hr$$

Step 4: COMPUTE.

$$\frac{\overset{12}{(DD)} \mid \overset{80}{(KG)} \mid (60) \mid \overset{100}{(VOL)}}{\mid \mid \underset{1000\,\mathbf{000}}{(DRUG)}} = \boxed{5.8 \; cc/hr}$$

**7.22** An angina patient is receiving nitroglycerin at 5 cc/hr. The pharmacy mixed the drip and you note the 300 cc D5W IV bag to have 75 mg of nitroglycerin in it. Your patient is 121 kg. What dose is the patient receiving?

Step 1: Write out the blank template.

$$\frac{\text{(DD)} \mid \text{(KG)} \mid \text{(60)} \mid \text{(VOL)}}{\text{(DRUG)}} = \text{cc/hr}$$

Step 2: Identify anatomy and assign values to the template.
Keep the '60' term for "per min" drugs and keep the KG if it is weight based.

$$\frac{\text{X} \quad\quad\quad\quad \checkmark \quad 300}{\text{(DD)} \mid \cancel{\text{(KG)}} \mid \text{(60)} \mid \frac{\text{(VOL)}}{\text{(DRUG)}}} = 5 \text{ cc/hr}$$
75

Step 3: Synchronize the dose and concentration by adding 3 zeros if the units do not match.

$$\frac{\text{X} \quad\quad\quad\quad \checkmark \quad 300}{\text{(DD)} \mid \cancel{\text{(KG)}} \mid \text{(60)} \mid \frac{\text{(VOL)}}{\text{(DRUG)}}} = 5 \text{ cc/hr}$$
75 **000**

Step 4: COMPUTE (Multiply, then Divide, Divide, ~~Divide~~).

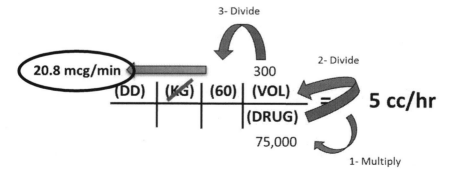

3- Divide

2- Divide

20.8 mcg/min

$$\frac{300}{\text{(DD)} \mid \cancel{\text{(KG)}} \mid \text{(60)} \mid \frac{\text{(VOL)}}{\text{(DRUG)}}} = 5 \text{ cc/hr}$$
75,000

1- Multiply

**7.23** Your septic patient is hypotensive. You choose Levophed and decide to administer 15 mcg/min. On hand you have 10 mg of drug, a 500 cc IV bag of NS, and a patient weighing 75 kg. What rate will you run this infusion at?

Step 1: Write out the blank template.

$$\frac{(DD) \mid (KG) \mid (60) \mid (VOL)}{\mid \quad \mid \quad \mid (DRUG)} = cc/hr$$

Step 2: Identify anatomy and assign values to the template.
Keep the '60' term for "per min" drugs and keep the KG if it is weight based.

$$\frac{\overset{15}{(DD)} \mid \overset{}{(\cancel{KG})} \mid (60) \mid \overset{500}{(VOL)}}{\mid \quad \mid \quad \mid \underset{10}{(DRUG)}} = \text{xxxx } cc/hr$$

Step 3: Synchronize the dose and concentration by adding
3 zeros if the units do not match.

$$\frac{\overset{15}{(DD)} \mid \overset{}{(\cancel{KG})} \mid (60) \mid \overset{500}{(VOL)}}{\mid \quad \mid \quad \mid \underset{10\ 000}{(DRUG)}} = \text{xxxx } cc/hr$$

Step 4: COMPUTE.

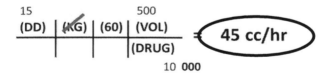

$$\frac{\overset{15}{(DD)} \mid \overset{}{(\cancel{KG})} \mid (60) \mid \overset{500}{(VOL)}}{\mid \quad \mid \quad \mid \underset{10\ 000}{(DRUG)}} = \boxed{45\ cc/hr}$$

**7.24** Your patient with 2nd degree heart block is receiving Isuprel at 400 cc/hr. The infusion bag looks to have 3 mg in 250 cc of NS. Your patient weighs 71 kg. What dose is the patient receiving? [Isuprel's dose units are mcg/kg/min]

Step 1: Write out the blank template.

$$\frac{(DD) \mid (KG) \mid (60) \mid (VOL)}{\mid \qquad \mid \qquad \mid (DRUG)} = cc/hr$$

Step 2: Identify anatomy and assign values to the template.
Keep the '60' term for "per min" drugs and keep the KG if it is weight based.

$$\frac{\overset{X}{(DD)} \mid \overset{71}{(KG)} \mid \overset{\checkmark}{(60)} \mid \overset{250}{(VOL)}}{\mid \qquad \mid \qquad \mid \underset{3}{(DRUG)}} = 100 \ cc/hr$$

Step 3: Synchronize the dose and concentration by adding
     3 zeros if the units do not match.

$$\frac{\overset{X}{(DD)} \mid \overset{71}{(KG)} \mid \overset{\checkmark}{(60)} \mid \overset{250}{(VOL)}}{\mid \qquad \mid \qquad \mid (DRUG)}_{3\,000} = 100 \ cc/hr$$

Step 4: COMPUTE (Multiply, then Divide, Divide, Divide).

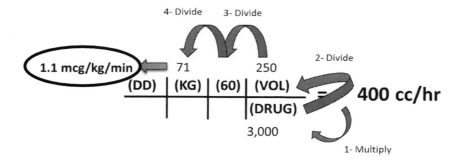

**7.25** Dobutamine needs to be administered to a heart failure patient. You have a vial of 500 mg of dobutamine and a 250 cc IV bag of NS. The patient weighs 97 kg. You decide to administer 7 mcg/kg/min. What rate will you run this infusion at?

Step 1: Write out the blank template.

$$\frac{(DD) \mid (KG) \mid (60) \mid (VOL)}{\mid \quad \mid \quad \mid (DRUG)} = cc/hr$$

Step 2: Identify anatomy and assign values to the template.
Keep the '60' term for "per min" drugs and keep the KG if it is weight based.

$$\frac{\overset{7}{(DD)} \mid \overset{97}{(KG)} \mid (60) \mid \overset{250}{(VOL)}}{\mid \quad \mid \quad \mid \underset{500}{(DRUG)}} = xxxx \ cc/hr$$

Step 3: Synchronize the dose and concentration by adding 3 zeros if the units do not match.

$$\frac{\overset{7}{(DD)} \mid \overset{97}{(KG)} \mid (60) \mid \overset{250}{(VOL)}}{\mid \quad \mid \quad \mid \underset{500 \ \mathbf{000}}{(DRUG)}} = xxxx \ cc/hr$$

Step 4: COMPUTE.

$$\frac{\overset{7}{(DD)} \mid \overset{97}{(KG)} \mid (60) \mid \overset{250}{(VOL)}}{\mid \quad \mid \quad \mid \underset{500 \ \mathbf{000}}{(DRUG)}} = \boxed{20.4 \ cc/hr}$$

73

**7.26** A patient requires a heparin infusion and has already received the bolus. The MD is asking for 800 units/h. Your patient is 100 kg. A nurse in the room suggests the correct rate to be 80cc/hr. (1) What rate will you run this infusion at? (2) Is the nurse correct?

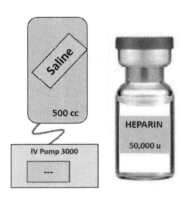

Step 1: Write out the blank template.

$$\frac{(DD) \mid (KG) \mid (60) \mid (VOL)}{\mid \mid (DRUG)} = cc/hr$$

Step 2: Identify anatomy and assign values to the template.
Keep the '60' term for "per min" drugs and keep the KG if it is weight based.

$$\frac{800 \qquad\qquad 500}{(DD) \mid \cancel{(KG)} \mid \cancel{(60)} \mid (VOL)}{\mid \mid (DRUG)} = xxxx \ cc/hr$$
$$50,000$$

Step 3: Synchronize the dose and concentration by adding 3 zeros if the units do not match.

$$\frac{800 \qquad\qquad 500}{(DD) \mid \cancel{(KG)} \mid \cancel{(60)} \mid (VOL)}{\mid \mid (DRUG)} = xxxx \ cc/hr$$
$$50,000 \qquad \textbf{No zeros needed}$$

Step 4: COMPUTE.

$$\frac{800 \qquad\qquad 500}{(DD) \mid \cancel{(KG)} \mid \cancel{(60)} \mid (VOL)}{\mid \mid (DRUG)} = \boxed{8 \ cc/hr}$$
$$50,000 \qquad \textbf{No zeros needed}$$

The nurse is wrong by a magnitude of 10 and the patient would be receiving way too high of a dose of heparin.

**7.27** A diabetic patient needs to be administered insulin via continuous infusion. Pharmacy delivers an infusion bag as pictured below. The physician orders 7 u/hr for this 91 kg patient. You observe the IV pump running at the rate below. Is this the correct infusion rate? If not, how would you correct it?

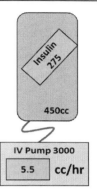

Step 1: Write out the blank template.

$$\frac{(DD) \mid (KG) \mid (60) \mid (VOL)}{\mid \mid (DRUG)} = cc/hr$$

Step 2: Identify anatomy and assign values to the template.
Keep the '60' term for "per min" drugs and keep the KG if it is weight based.

IV Pump 3000

| 5.5 | cc/hr |

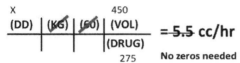

$$\frac{X \qquad\qquad 450}{(DD) \mid (\cancel{KG}) \mid (\cancel{60}) \mid (VOL)}{\mid \mid (DRUG)} = 5.5 \ cc/hr$$
275

Step 3: Synchronize the dose and concentration by adding 3 zeros if the units do not match.

$$\frac{X \qquad\qquad 450}{(DD) \mid (\cancel{KG}) \mid (\cancel{60}) \mid (VOL)}{\mid \mid (DRUG)} = 5.5 \ cc/hr$$
275        **No zeros needed**

Step 4: COMPUTE (Multiply, then Divide, Divide, ~~Divide~~).

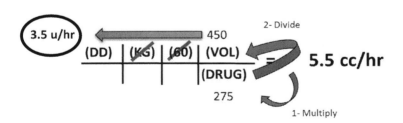

2- Divide

3.5 u/hr

450

$$\frac{(DD) \mid (\cancel{KG}) \mid (\cancel{60}) \mid (VOL)}{\mid \mid (DRUG)}$$

275

= 5.5 cc/hr

1- Multiply

The current rate (5.5 cc/hr) is only delivering a dose of 3.5 u/hr. So, because of the ratio relationship between dose and rate, if we double the rate to 11 cc/hr the new dosage would be 7 u/hr on the nose.

**7.28** A hypotensive patient has a neosynepherine drip running at 3 cc/hr. You note the 250 cc infusion bag to contain 1 mg of drug. The patient is 70 kg. The medical staff reports the medication is infusing at 10 mcg/min. Is the patient receiving the correct dose? If not, how would you correct it?

Step 1: Write out the blank template.

$$\frac{(DD) \mid (KG) \mid (60) \mid (VOL)}{\mid \mid (DRUG)} = cc/hr$$

Step 2: Identify anatomy and assign values to the template.
Keep the '60' term for "per min" drugs and keep the KG if it is weight based.

$$\frac{\overset{X}{(DD)} \mid \cancel{(KG)} \mid (60) \mid \overset{250}{(VOL)}}{\mid \mid \underset{1}{(DRUG)}} = 3\ cc/hr$$

Step 3: Synchronize the dose and concentration by adding 3 zeros if the units do not match.

$$\frac{\overset{X}{(DD)} \mid \cancel{(KG)} \mid (60) \mid \overset{250}{(VOL)}}{\mid \mid (DRUG)} = 3\ cc/hr$$

1  **000**

Step 4: COMPUTE (Multiply, then Divide, Divide, ~~Divide~~).

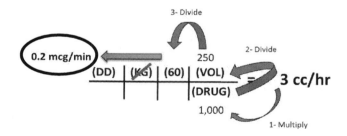

The current rate (3 cc/hr) is only delivering a dose of 0.2 mcg/min. To get 0.2 to equal 10 , we'd have to multiply it by 50. Therefore, Multiply the rate by 50. Changing the rate to 150 cc/hr (50 x 3 cc/hr) would change the dose delivered to 10 mcg/min.

**7.29** A patient you are caring for needs to be administered an infusion of nipride at 5 mcg/kg/min. The patient weighs 85 kg. You have 50 mg of nipride available and a 250 cc IV bag. What rate will you run this infusion at? An app on your phone indicates the rate should be 130 cc/hr. Is the app correct?

Step 1: Write out the blank template.

$$\frac{(DD) \mid (KG) \mid (60) \mid (VOL)}{\mid \quad \mid \quad \mid (DRUG)} = cc/hr$$

Step 2: Identify anatomy and assign values to the template.
Keep the '60' term for "per min" drugs and keep the KG if it is weight based.

$$\frac{\overset{5}{(DD)} \mid \overset{85}{(KG)} \mid (60) \mid \overset{250}{(VOL)}}{\mid \quad \mid \quad \mid \underset{50}{(DRUG)}} = xxxx \ \textbf{cc/hr}$$

Step 3: Synchronize the dose and concentration by adding 3 zeros if the units do not match.

$$\frac{\overset{5}{(DD)} \mid \overset{85}{(KG)} \mid (60) \mid \overset{250}{(VOL)}}{\mid \quad \mid \quad \mid \underset{50\ 000}{(DRUG)}} = xxxx \ \textbf{cc/hr}$$

Step 4: COMPUTE.

$$\frac{\overset{5}{(DD)} \mid \overset{85}{(KG)} \mid (60) \mid \overset{250}{(VOL)}}{\mid \quad \mid \quad \mid \underset{50\ 000}{(DRUG)}} = \boxed{127.5 \ \textbf{cc/hr}}$$

The app is very close, but not exact. Here every 127.5 cc/hr gets you another 5 mcg/kg/min. So if you wanted to deliver 10 mcg/kg/min, simply double the rate (255 cc/hr).

**7.30** A patient is in shock and you need to administer epinephrine. You will administer 6 mcg/ min. You have epi on hand as pictured below. The patient is 81 kg. After examining some drug tables, your partner suggests a rate of 3 cc/hr. Is he correct?

Step 1: Write out the blank template.

$$\frac{(DD) \mid (KG) \mid (60) \mid (VOL)}{\mid \quad \mid \quad \mid (DRUG)} = cc/hr$$

Step 2: Identify anatomy and assign values to the template.
Keep the '60' term for "per min" drugs and keep the KG if it is weight based.

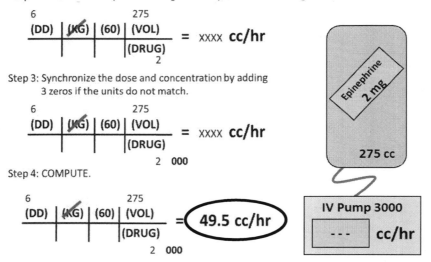

Step 3: Synchronize the dose and concentration by adding 3 zeros if the units do not match.

Step 4: COMPUTE.

No, your partner is way off. To deliver 6 mcg/min of epi at the above concentration, the IV pump needs to be set to deliver 49.5 cc/hr. If you wanted to double the dose, simply double the rate.

**7.31** You are transporting a patient currently receiving dobutamine at a rate of 25 cc/hr. The IV bag which was mixed by their pharmacy has a label that reads as pictured below. The patient weight is 101 kg. What dose is the patient receiving? The sending medical staff reports the patient is receiving 9 mcg/kg/min. Is the patient receiving the correct dose? If not, how would you correct it?

Step 1: Write out the blank template.

$$\frac{(DD) \mid (KG) \mid (60) \mid (VOL)}{\mid \quad \mid \quad \mid (DRUG)} = cc/hr$$

Dobutamine
500 mg

470 cc

Step 2: Identify anatomy and assign values to the template. Keep the '60' term for "per min" drugs and keep the KG if it is weight based.

$$\frac{X \quad 101 \quad \checkmark \quad 470}{(DD) \mid (KG) \mid (60) \mid (VOL)} = 25\ cc/hr$$
$$\frac{}{\mid \quad \mid \quad \mid (DRUG)\ 500}$$

IV Pump 3000

| 25 | cc/hr |

Step 3: Synchronize the dose and concentration by adding 3 zeros if the units do not match.

$$\frac{X \quad 101 \quad \checkmark \quad 470}{(DD) \mid (KG) \mid (60) \mid (VOL)} = 25cc/hr$$
$$\frac{}{\mid \quad \mid \quad \mid (DRUG)\ 500\ \mathbf{000}}$$

Step 4: COMPUTE (Multiply, then Divide, Divide, Divide).

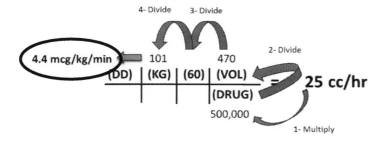

4- Divide    3- Divide

2- Divide

4.4 mcg/kg/min    101    470
(DD) | (KG) | (60) | (VOL)    =    25 cc/hr
              | (DRUG)
              500,000

1- Multiply

No, the patient is only receiving 4.4 mcg/kg/min. By doubling the rate, you'd be very close to the 9 mcg/kg/min.

**7.32** A stroke patient is in your care and propofol is chosen for continued sedation. You decide to start with 15 mcg/kg/min. The bottle comes with 1000 mg in 100 cc. The patient weighs 91 kg. Your partner thinks the IV pump should be set to 8 cc/hr. Is your partner correct? If not, what can be done to correct it?

Step 1: Write out the blank template.

$$\frac{(DD) \mid (KG) \mid (60) \mid (VOL)}{\mid \quad \mid \quad \mid (DRUG)} = cc/hr$$

Step 2: Identify anatomy and assign values to the template. Keep the '60' term for "per min" drugs and keep the KG if it is weight based.

$$\frac{\overset{15}{(DD)} \mid \overset{91}{(KG)} \mid (60) \mid \overset{100}{(VOL)}}{\mid \quad \mid \quad \mid \underset{1000}{(DRUG)}} = \text{xxxx } cc/hr$$

Step 3: Synchronize the dose and concentration by adding 3 zeros if the units do not match.

$$\frac{\overset{15}{(DD)} \mid \overset{91}{(KG)} \mid (60) \mid \overset{100}{(VOL)}}{\mid \quad \mid \quad \mid \underset{1000\,000}{(DRUG)}} = \text{xxxx } cc/hr$$

Step 4: COMPUTE.

$$\frac{\overset{15}{(DD)} \mid \overset{91}{(KG)} \mid (60) \mid \overset{100}{(VOL)}}{\mid \quad \mid \quad \mid \underset{1000\,000}{(DRUG)}} = \boxed{8.2 \ cc/hr}$$

Your partner is correct, and only off by 0.2 in this case.

**7.33** Labetalol has been chosen for your hypertensive emergency patient. See below for the quantities available. Your patient weighs 84 kg. You decide to begin the dose at 4 mg/min. You first calculated the needed infusion rate as 60 cc/hr, but you feel this may be high. Is your suspicion warranted, or was your original calculation correct?

Step 1: Write out the blank template.

$$\frac{(DD) \mid (KG) \mid (60) \mid (VOL)}{\mid \mid (DRUG)} = cc/hr$$

Step 2: Identify anatomy and assign values to the template. Keep the '60' term for "per min" drugs and keep the KG if it is weight based.

$$\frac{\overset{4}{(DD)} \mid \overset{}{(\cancel{KG})} \mid (60) \mid \overset{250}{(VOL)}}{\mid \mid \underset{1}{(DRUG)}} = xxxx \ cc/hr$$

Step 3: Synchronize the dose and concentration by adding 3 zeros if the units do not match.

$$\frac{\overset{4}{(DD)} \mid \overset{}{(\cancel{KG})} \mid (60) \mid \overset{250}{(VOL)}}{\mid \mid \underset{1\ 000}{(DRUG)}} = xxxx \ cc/hr$$

Step 4: COMPUTE.

$$\frac{\overset{4}{(DD)} \mid \overset{}{(\cancel{KG})} \mid (60) \mid \overset{250}{(VOL)}}{\mid \mid \underset{1\ 000}{(DRUG)}} = \boxed{60 \ cc/hr}$$

Your original calculation was correct. You must have been practicing with a really reliable method. Cool trick: divide both dose and rate by 4. This results in 1 mg/min per every 15 cc/hr. This means if you wanted to increase the dose to 5 mg/min, simply add 15 cc/hr to the current infusion rate. Check the math: 75 cc/hr gets you 5 mg/min.

**7.34** Your patient is receiving a continuous infusion of neosynepherine as pictured as below. The patient is 72 kg. You have injected 10 mg into a 250 cc NS IV bag. It is reported that the patient is receiving a dose of 18 mcg/min. Is this correct? If not, how would you correct it?

Step 1: Write out the blank template.

$$\frac{(DD) \mid (KG) \mid (60) \mid (VOL)}{\mid \quad \mid \quad \mid (DRUG)} = cc/hr$$

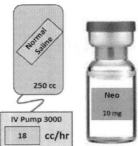

Step 2: Identify anatomy and assign values to the template. Keep the '60' term for "per min" drugs and keep the KG if it is weight based.

$$\frac{(DD) \mid (\cancel{KG}) \mid (60)^{\checkmark} \mid (VOL)^{250}}{\mid \quad \mid \quad \mid (DRUG)_{10}} = 18 \ cc/hr$$

Step 3: Synchronize the dose and concentration by addin̨ 3 zeros if the units do not match.

$$\frac{(DD) \mid (\cancel{KG}) \mid (60)^{\checkmark} \mid (VOL)^{250}}{\mid \quad \mid \quad \mid (DRUG)} = 18 \ cc/hr$$
10 000

Step 4: COMPUTE (Multiply, then Divide, Divide, ~~Divide~~).

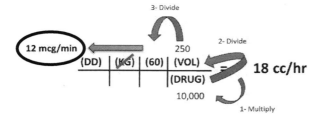

It is not correct, but it is close. This requires a small tweak. The patient is receiving 12 mcg/min, and the order was for 10. Divide both dose and rate by 12 (the value of the dose). This results in 1 mcg/min per every 1.5 cc/hr. Therefore, to get to 10 mcg/min, reduce the rate by 3 cc/hr. This would yield a dose of 10 mcg/min.

# 8 SHIFT PRACTICE SESSIONS

By now, you should be feeling pretty damn good. You should feel that way. You've tackled a monster and defeated it. Now it's time to begin perfecting and maintaining this skill. The following sheets are designed in the format of a daily calculation devotional called sessions. Each session has 3 problems. Each day for your shift you should complete the 3 problems before your first call or patient, if possible. This will prime you for any calculation problem you'll face. In a year's time, you'll be beyond a Calc Hero.

NOTE: Rounding can sometimes be subjective. I have rounded to the nearest tenth's place using the indigenous iPhone calculator app. If you see one that is terribly off let us know by scanning the QR code on the Table of Contents page and we will fix it. We have taken extra care to ensure your experience with this text is a positive one, so if you see something weird, let us know.

Date: _____

A patient requires a heparin infusion and has already received the bolus. The MD is asking for 800 units/h. The pre-mixed bag is supplied with 50,000 units in 500 cc of D5W. Your patient is 100 kg. What rate will you run this infusion at?

A hypotensive patient has a neosynepherine drip running at 3 cc/hr. You note the 250 cc infusion bag to contain 1 mg of drug. The patient is 70 kg. What dose is the patient receiving?

A diabetic patient needs to be administered insulin via continuous infusion. Pharmacy delivers an infusion bag with 300 units in 275 cc of NS. The physician orders 9 u/hr for this 85 kg patient. What rate will you run this infusion at?

## SHIFT 2

Date: _____

A patient you are caring for needs to be administered an infusion of nipride at 5 mcg/kg/min. The patient weighs 71 kg. You have 35 mg of nipride available and a 250 cc IV bag. What rate will you run this infusion at?

A patient is in shock and you need to administer epinephrine. You will administer 3 mcg/ min. Your plan is to mix 1 mg of 1:1000 epi into a 500 cc IV bag. The patient is 61 kg. What rate will you run this infusion at?

You are transporting a patient currently receiving dobutamine at a rate of 13 cc/hr. The 500 cc IV bag has a label that reads "350 mg of dobutamine". The patient weight is 92 kg. What dose is the patient receiving?

# SHIFT 3

Date: _____

A neuro patient is in your care and propofol is chosen for continued sedation. You decide to start with 8 mcg/kg/min. The bottle comes with 1000 mg in 100 cc. The patient weighs 71 kg. What rate will you run this infusion at?

Labetalol has been chosen for your hypertensive emergency patient. You have 1 gram available and will use a 500 cc IV bag. Your patient weighs 95 kg. You decide to begin the dose at 2 mg/min. What rate will you run this infusion at?

Amiodarone is infusing for a patient with SVT at 17 cc/hr. The sending facility has provided you with a 500 cc D5W containing 900 mg of amiodarone. The patient weighs 96 kg. What dose is the patient receiving?

# SHIFT 4

Date: _____

---

Heparin 20,000 units in 450 mL D5W is ordered to run at 1,200 units/hour. The patient is 104 kg. What rate will you run this infusion at?

---

A MD wants you to continue a fentanyl drip for an intubated cancer patient targeting 250 mcg/hr. Three (3) mg of fentanyl was injected into a 325 cc D5W IV bag. The patient weighs 87 kg. What rate will you run this infusion at?

---

You patient requires sedation while on the mechanical ventilator, and you decide to administer propofol. On hand, you have a glass bottle with 1000 mg dissolved into a 100 cc lipid emulsion. You decide to start the infusion at 12 mcg/kg/hr. The patient is 80 kg. What rate will you run this infusion at?

## SHIFT 5

Date: _____

A patient is receiving a lidocaine drip. The order is for 2 mg per minute. One gram of lidocaine has been added to a 250 mL IV bag. The patient weighs 93 kg. What rate will you run this infusion at?

You need to administer insulin to your DKA patient and decide 4 u/hr is needed. The patient weighs 59 kg. Pharmacy has prepared for you an IV bag of 250 NS with 85 units injected into it. What rate will you run this infusion at?

An angina patient is receiving nitroglycerin at 5 cc/hr. The pharmacy mixed the drip and you note the 300 cc D5W IV bag to have 75 mg of nitroglycerin in it. Your patient is 121 kg. What dose is the patient receiving?

# SHIFT 6

Date: _____

A hypotensive patient requires norepinephrine. On hand, you have 4 mg and 250 cc of NS. You wish to administer 15 mcg/min. The patient weighs 82 kg. What rate will you run this infusion at?

A patient with a pulmonary embolus is receiving streptokinase. The protocol states 500k IU should be injected into a 250 cc bag of NS and be delivered at 125k IU/hr. Your patient weighs 71 kg. What rate will you run this infusion at?

Your septic patient is hypotensive. You choose Levophed and decide to administer 15 mcg/min. On hand you have 10 mg of drug, a 500 cc IV bag of NS, and a patient weighing 75 kg. What rate will you run this infusion at?

# SHIFT 7

Date: _____

A patient requires Brevibloc for tachycardia. The order calls for 45 mcg/kg/min. On hand, you have 950 mg in 250 cc of D5W. The patient weighs 82 kg. What rate will you run this infusion at?

Amiodarone is infusing for a patient with SVT at 14 cc/hr. The sending facility has provided you with a 250 cc D5W containing 750 mg of amiodarone. The patient weighs 101 kg. What dose is the patient receiving? [Hint: Amiodarone is in mg/min].

Your patient with 2nd degree heart block is receiving isuprel at 100 cc/hr. The infusion bag looks to have 3 mg in 250 cc of NS. Your patient weighs 71 kg. What dose is the patient receiving? [Hint: Isuprel is in mcg/min].

# SHIFT 8

Date: _____

---

An angina patient is receiving nitroglycerin at 3 cc/hr. The pharmacy mixed the drip and you note the 250 cc D5W IV bag to have 58 mg of nitroglycerin in it. Your patient is 92 kg. What dose is the patient receiving?

---

Your septic patient is hypotensive. You choose Levophed and decide to administer 11 mcg/min. On hand you have 8 mg of drug, a 250 cc IV bag of NS, and a patient weighing 80 kg. What rate will you run this infusion at?

---

Doubutamine needs to be administered to a heart failure patient. You have a vial of 500 mg of dobutamine and a 250 cc IV bag of NS. The patient weighs 97 kg. You decide to administer 7 mcg/kg/min. What rate will you run this infusion at?

## SHIFT 9

Date: _____

A diabetic patient needs to be administered insulin via continuous infusion. Pharmacy delivers an infusion bag with 300 units in 275 cc of NS. The physician orders 9 u/hr for this 85 kg patient. What rate will you run this infusion at?

A patient requires a heparin infusion and has already received the bolus. The MD is asking for 800 units/h. The pre-mixed bag is supplied with 50,000 units in 500 cc of D5W. Your patient is 100 kg. A nurse in the room suggests the correct rate to be 15 cc/hr. Is this correct? If not, how would you correct it?

A diabetic patient needs to be administered insulin via continuous infusion. Pharmacy delivers an infusion bag with 275 units in 450 cc of NS. The physician orders 7 u/hr for this 91 kg patient, and you observe the IV pump running at 5.5 u/hr. Is this the correct infusion rate? If not, how would you correct it?

## SHIFT 10

Date: _____

---

A hypotensive patient has a neosynepherine drip running at 5 cc/hr. You note the 500 cc infusion bag to contain 1 mg of drug. The patient is 55 kg. The medical staff reports the medication is infusing at 10 mcg/min. Is the patient receiving the correct dose? If not, how would you correct it??

---

A patient you are caring for needs to be administered an infusion of nipride at 4 mcg/kg/min. The patient weighs 75 kg. You have 25 mg of nipride available and a 150 cc IV bag. What rate will you run this infusion at? An app on your phone indicates the rate should be 50 cc/hr. Is the app correct?

---

A patient is in shock and you need to administer epinephrine. You will administer 6 mcg/ min. Your plan is to mix 2 mg of 1:1000 epi into a 275 cc IV bag. The patient is 81 kg. After examining some drug tables, your partner suggests a rate of 16 cc/hr. Is he correct?

## SHIFT 11

Date: _____

A patient requires a heparin infusion and has already received the bolus. The MD is asking for 800 units/h. The pre-mixed bag is supplied with 50,000 units in 500 cc of D5W. Your patient is 100 kg. What rate will you run this infusion at?

Dopamine is being infused to a hypotensive patient at 15 cc/hr. The patient is 75 kg. Pharmacy has mixed the 500 cc NS IV bag with 1000 mg. What dose is the patient receiving?

A hypotensive patient has a neosynepherine drip running at 8 cc/hr. You note the 250 cc infusion bag to contain 1 mg of drug. The patient is 95 kg. The medical staff reports the medication is infusing at 10 mcg/min. Is the patient receiving the correct dose? If not, how would you correct it?

# SHIFT 12

Date: _____

---

Amiodarone is infusing for a patient with SVT at 15 cc/hr. The sending facility has provided you with a 250 cc D5W containing 750 mg of amiodarone. The patient weighs 82 kg. What dose is the patient receiving?

---

A patient is receiving a lidocaine drip. The order is for 5 mg per minute. One gram of lidocaine has been added to a 250 mL IV bag. The patient weighs 71 kg. What rate will you run this infusion at?

---

A stroke patient is in your care and propofol is chosen for continued sedation. You decide to start with 9 mcg/kg/min. The bottle comes with 1000 mg in 100 cc. The patient weighs 75 kg. Your partner thinks the IV pump should be set to 10 cc/hr. Is your partner correct? If not, what can be done to correct it?

Date: _____

---

Labetalol has been chosen for your hypertensive emergency patient. You have 1 gram available and will use a 500 cc IV bag. Your patient weighs 95 kg. You decide to begin the dose at 4 mg/min. What rate will you run this infusion at?

---

A hypotensive patient requires norepinephrine. On hand, you have 7 mg and 250 cc of NS. You wish to administer 27 mcg/min. The patient weighs 82 kg. What rate will you run this infusion at?

---

A patient requires a heparin infusion and has already received the bolus. The MD is asking for 750 units/h. The pre-mixed bag is supplied with 50,000 units in 250 cc of D5W. Your patient is 87 kg. A nurse in the room suggests the correct rate to be 12 cc/hr. Is this correct? If not, how would you correct it?

# SHIFT 14

Date: _____

Norepinephrine is being run at 11 cc/hr. The IV bag reads 5 mg in 500 of normal saline. The patient weighs 85 kg. What dose is the patient receiving?

Dopamine is being infused to a hypotensive patient at 12 cc/hr. The patient is 81 kg. Pharmacy has mixed the 250 cc NS IV bag with 1000 mg. What dose is the patient receiving?

You are transporting a patient currently receiving dobutamine at a rate of 30 cc/hr. The IV bag has 500 mg in 250 cc D5W. The patient weight is 85 kg. What dose is the patient receiving? The sending medical staff reports the patient is receiving 12 mcg/kg/min. Is the patient receiving the correct dose? If not, how would you correct it?

## SHIFT 15

Date: _____

A hypotensive patient has a neosynepherine drip running at 5 cc/hr. You note the 500 cc infusion bag to contain 1 mg of drug. The patient is 50 kg. What dose is the patient receiving?

You need to administer insulin to your DKA patient and decide 6 u/hr is needed. The patient weighs 91 kg. Pharmacy has prepared for you an IV bag of 325 NS with 90 units injected into it. What rate will you run this infusion at?

A diabetic patient needs to be administered insulin via continuous infusion. Pharmacy delivers an infusion bag with 300 units in 500 cc of NS. The physician orders 8 u/hr for this 84 kg patient, and you observe the IV pump running at 9 cc/hr. Is this the correct infusion rate? If not, how would you correct it?

# SHIFT 16

Date: _____

Heparin 20,000 units in 500 mL D5W is ordered to run at 1,500 units/hour. The patient is 70 kg. What rate will you run this infusion at?

Amiodarone is infusing for a patient with SVT at 12 cc/hr. The sending facility has provided you with a 250 cc D5W containing 750 mg of amiodarone. The patient weighs 82 kg. What dose is the patient receiving?

A patient is in shock and you need to administer epinephrine. You will administer 9 mcg/ min. Your plan is to mix 1 mg of 1:1000 epi into a 250 cc IV bag. The patient is 65 kg. After examining some drug tables, your partner suggests a rate of 5 cc/hr. Is he correct?

## SHIFT 17

Date: _____

A diabetic patient needs to be administered insulin via continuous infusion. Pharmacy delivers an infusion bag with 300 units in 275 cc of NS. The physician orders 9 u/hr for this 85 kg patient. What rate will you run this infusion at?

Norepinephrine is being run at 13 cc/hr. The IV bag reads 3 mg in 250 of normal saline. The patient weighs 95 kg. What dose is the patient receiving?

A patient you are caring for needs to be administered an infusion of nipride at 2 mcg/kg/min. The patient weighs 95 kg. You have 50 mg of nipride available and a 250 cc IV bag. What rate will you run this infusion at? An app on your phone indicates the rate should be 60 cc/hr. Is the app correct?

# SHIFT 18

Date: _____

---

A patient is receiving a lidocaine drip. The order is for 3 mg per minute. One gram of lidocaine has been added to a 500 mL IV bag. The patient weighs 110 kg. What rate will you run this infusion at?

---

Your patient with 2nd degree heart block is receiving isuprel at 100 cc/hr. The infusion bag looks to have 3 mg in 250 cc of NS. Your patient weighs 71 kg. What dose is the patient receiving?

---

Labetalol has been chosen for your hypertensive emergency patient. You have 1 gram available and will use a 250 cc IV bag. Your patient weighs 84 kg. You decide to begin the dose at 4 mg/min. You first calculated the needed infusion rate as 60 cc/hr, but you feel this may be high. Is your suspicion warranted, or was your original calculation correct?

# SHIFT 19

Date: _____

---

A patient is in shock and you need to administer epinephrine. You will administer 7 mcg/ min. Your plan is to mix 1 mg of 1:1000 epi into a 500 cc IV bag. The patient is 65 kg. What rate will you run this infusion at?

---

Nipride is being delivered at 42 cc/hr. The patient weighs 75 kg. On hand, you have 50 mg of Nipride in a 250 cc glass bottle of 0.9% saline. What dose is the patient receiving?

---

You are transporting a patient currently receiving dobutamine at a rate of 21 cc/hr. The IV bag which was mixed by their pharmacy has 427 mg in 320 of D5W. The patient weight is 85 kg. What dose is the patient receiving? The sending medical staff reports the patient is receiving 12 mcg/kg/min. Is the patient receiving the correct dose? If not, how would you correct it?

# SHIFT 20

Date: _____

---

A MD wants you to continue a fentanyl drip for an intubated cancer patient targeting 200 mcg/hr. Six (6) mg of fentanyl was injected into a 250 cc D5W IV bag. The patient weighs 85 kg. What rate will you run this infusion at?

---

A patient requires Brevibloc for tachycardia. The order calls for 35 mcg/kg/min. On hand, you have 1250 mg in 250 cc of D5W. The patient weighs 99 kg. What rate will you run this infusion at?

---

Your patient is receiving a continuous infusion of neosynepherine at 22 cc/hr. The patient is 80 kg. You have injected 15 mg into a 250 cc NS IV bag. It is reported that the patient is receiving a dose of 13 mcg/min. Is this correct? If not, how would you correct it?

Date: _____

A patient you are caring for needs to be administered an infusion of nipride at 5 mcg/kg/min. The patient weighs 88 kg. You have 25 mg of nipride available and a 500 cc IV bag. What rate will you run this infusion at?

A patient with a pulmonary embolus is receiving streptokinase. The protocol states 555k IU should be injected into a 250 cc bag of NS and be delivered at 100k IU/hr. Your patient weighs 98 kg. What rate will you run this infusion at?

A patient requires a heparin infusion and has already received the bolus. The MD is asking for 500 units/h. The pre-mixed bag is supplied with 50,000 units in 250 cc of D5W. Your patient is 78 kg. A nurse in the room suggests the correct rate to be 21 cc/hr. Is this correct? If not, how would you correct it?

# SHIFT 22

Date: _____

---

The IV pump reads "23 cc/hr". Your patient is receiving a continuous infusion of neosynepherine. You have injected 10 mg into a 250 cc NS IV bag. The patient is 75 kg. What dose is the patient receiving?

---

An angina patient is receiving nitroglycerin at 8 cc/hr. The pharmacy mixed the drip and you note the 250 cc D5W IV bag to have 100 mg of nitroglycerin in it. Your patient is 84 kg. What dose is the patient receiving?

---

A stroke patient is in your care and propofol is chosen for continued sedation. You decide to start with 11 mcg/kg/min. The bottle comes with 1000 mg in 100 cc. The patient weighs 88 kg. Your partner thinks the IV pump should be set to 20 cc/hr. Is your partner correct? If not, what can be done to correct it?

Date: _____

Your septic patient is hypotensive. You choose Levophed and decide to administer 21 mcg/min. On hand you have 10 mg of drug, a 250 cc IV bag of NS, and a patient weighing 100 kg. What rate will you run this infusion at?

You are transporting a patient currently receiving dobutamine at a rate of 25 cc/hr. The 250 cc IV bag has a label that reads "500 mg of dobutamine". The patient weight is 77 kg. What dose is the patient receiving?

A diabetic patient needs to be administered insulin via continuous infusion. Pharmacy delivers an infusion bag with 250 units in 250 cc of NS. The physician orders 10 u/hr for this 70 kg patient, and you observe the IV pump running at 8 u/hr. Is this the correct infusion rate? If not, how would you correct it?

# SHIFT 24

Date: _____

---

A patient is receiving a lidocaine drip. The order is for 4 mg per minute. One gram of lidocaine has been added to a 250 mL IV bag. The patient weighs 100 kg. What rate will you run this infusion at?

---

A neuro patient is in your care and propofol is chosen for continued sedation. You decide to start with 8 mcg/kg/min. The bottle comes with 1000 mg in 100 cc. The patient weighs 55 kg. What rate will you run this infusion at?

---

A patient is in shock and you need to administer epinephrine. You will administer 10 mcg/ min. Your plan is to mix 1 mg of 1:1000 epi into a 500 cc IV bag. The patient is 98 kg. After examining some drug tables, your partner suggests a rate of 10 cc/hr. Is he correct?

**SHIFT 25**

Date: _____

A hypotensive patient requires norepinephrine. On hand, you have 9 mg and 400 cc of NS. You wish to administer 18 mcg/min. The patient weighs 62 kg. What rate will you run this infusion at?

You patient requires sedation while on the mechanical ventilator, and you decide to administer propofol. On hand, you have a glass bottle with 1000 mg dissolved into a 100 cc lipid emulsion. You decide to start the infusion at 15 mcg/kg/min. The patient is 90 kg. What rate will you run this infusion at?

A patient you are caring for needs to be administered an infusion of nipride at 5 mcg/kg/min. The patient weighs 79 kg. You have 50 mg of nipride available and a 500 cc IV bag. What rate will you run this infusion at? An app on your phone indicates the rate should be 50 cc/hr. Is the app correct?

# SHIFT 26

Date: _____

---

Your patient requires sedation while on the mechanical ventilator, and you decide to administer propofol. On hand, you have a glass bottle with 1000 mg dissolved into a 100 cc lipid emulsion. You decide to start the infusion at 25 mcg/kg/min. The patient is 101 kg. What rate will you run this infusion at?

---

Dobutamine needs to be administered to a heart failure patient. You have a vial of 250 mg of dobutamine and a 500 cc IV bag of NS. The patient weighs 85 kg. You decide to administer 11 mcg/kg/min. What rate will you run this infusion at?

---

Labetalol has been chosen for your hypertensive emergency patient. You have 1 gram available and will use a 500 cc IV bag. Your patient weighs 88 kg. You decide to begin the dose at 2 mg/min. You first calculated the needed infusion rate as 55 cc/hr, but you feel this may be high. Is your suspicion warranted, or was your original calculation correct?

## SHIFT 27

Date: _____

A patient with a pulmonary embolus is receiving streptokinase. The protocol states 550k IU should be injected into a 250 cc bag of NS and be delivered at 100k IU/hr. Your patient weighs 99 kg. What rate will you run this infusion at?

An angina patient is receiving nitroglycerin at 10 cc/hr. The pharmacy mixed the drip and you note the 250 cc D5W IV bag to have 100 mg of nitroglycerin in it. Your patient is 89 kg. What dose is the patient receiving?

Your patient is receiving a continuous infusion of neosynepherine at 23 cc/hr. The patient is 83 kg. You have injected 20 mg into a 250 cc NS IV bag. It is reported that the patient is receiving a dose of 15 mcg/min. Is this correct? If not, how would you correct it?

# SHIFT 28

Date: _____

Heparin 20,000 units in 250 mL D5W is ordered to run at 1,000 units/hour. The patient is 97 kg. What rate will you run this infusion at?

Your patient with 2nd degree heart block is receiving isuprel at 125 cc/hr. The infusion bag looks to have 5 mg in 500 cc of NS. Your patient weighs 60 kg. What dose is the patient receiving?

A stroke patient is in your care and propofol is chosen for continued sedation. You decide to start with 20 mcg/kg/min. The bottle comes with 1000 mg in 100 cc. The patient weighs 120 kg. Your partner thinks the IV pump should be set to 11 cc/hr. Is your partner correct? If not, what can be done to correct it?

# SHIFT 29

Date: _____

You need to administer insulin to your DKA patient and decide 7 u/hr is needed. The patient weighs 88 kg. Pharmacy has prepared for you an IV bag of 500 NS with 75 units injected into it. What rate will you run this infusion at?

Your septic patient is hypotensive. You choose Levophed and decide to administer 20 mcg/min. On hand you have 20 mg of drug, a 250 cc IV bag of NS, and a patient weighing 79 kg. What rate will you run this infusion at?

You are transporting a patient currently receiving dobutamine at a rate of 55 cc/hr. The IV bag which was mixed by their pharmacy has 400 mg in 280 NS. The patient weight is 85 kg. What dose is the patient receiving? The sending medical staff reports the patient is receiving 10 mcg/kg/min. Is the patient receiving the correct dose? If not, how would you correct it?

# SHIFT 30

Date: _____

A patient requires Brevibloc for tachycardia. The order calls for 50 mcg/kg/min. On hand, you have 1000 mg in 250 cc of D5W. The patient weighs 86 kg. What rate will you run this infusion at?

Dobutamine needs to be administered to a heart failure patient. You have a vial of 250 mg of dobutamine and a 500 cc IV bag of NS. The patient weighs 88 kg. You decide to administer 10 mcg/kg/min. What rate will you run this infusion at?

Labetalol has been chosen for your hypertensive emergency patient. You have 1 gram available and will use a 500 cc IV bag. Your patient weighs 97 kg. You decide to begin the dose at 3 mg/min. You first calculated the needed infusion rate as 50 cc/hr, but you feel this may be high. Is your suspicion warranted, or was your original calculation correct?

## SHIFT 31

Date: _____

A patient requires a heparin infusion and has already received the bolus. The MD is asking for 650 units/h. The pre-mixed bag is supplied with 50,000 units in 400 cc of D5W. Your patient is 90 kg. What rate will you run this infusion at?

A hypotensive patient has a neosynepherine drip running at 4 cc/hr. You note the 250 cc infusion bag to contain 2 mg of drug. The patient is 82 kg. What dose is the patient receiving?

A diabetic patient needs to be administered insulin via continuous infusion. Pharmacy delivers an infusion bag with 250 units in 275 cc of NS. The physician orders 10 u/hr for this 81 kg patient. What rate will you run this infusion at?

# SHIFT 32

Date: _____

A patient you are caring for needs to be administered an infusion of Nipride at 5 mcg/kg/min. The patient weighs 71 kg. You have 35 mg of Nipride available and a 250 cc IV bag. What rate will you run this infusion at?

A patient is in shock and you need to administer epinephrine. You will administer 3 mcg/ min. Your plan is to mix 1 mg of 1:1000 epi into a 500 cc IV bag. The patient is 61 kg. What rate will you run this infusion at?

You are transporting a patient currently receiving dobutamine at a rate of 13 cc/hr. The 500 cc IV bag has a label that reads "350 mg of dobutamine". The patient weight is 92 kg. What dose is the patient receiving?

**SHIFT 33**

Date: _____

A patient requires a heparin infusion and has already received the bolus. The MD is asking for 575 units/h. The pre-mixed bag is supplied with 50,000 units in 350 cc of D5W. Your patient is 101 kg. What rate will you run this infusion at?

A hypotensive patient has a neosynepherine drip running at 3 cc/hr. You note the 250 cc infusion bag to contain 1 mg of drug. The patient is 70 kg. What dose is the patient receiving?

A patient is in shock and you need to administer epinephrine. You will administer 9 mcg/ min. Your plan is to mix 1 mg of 1:1000 epi into a 250 cc IV bag. The patient is 65 kg. After examining some drug tables, your partner suggests a rate of 5 cc/hr. Is he correct?

# SHIFT 34

Date: _____

---

A patient requires a heparin infusion and has already received the bolus. The MD is asking for 700 units/h. The pre-mixed bag is supplied with 50,000 units in 250 cc of D5W. Your patient is 90 kg. What rate will you run this infusion at?

---

A hypotensive patient has a neosynepherine drip running at 5 cc/hr. You note the 500 cc infusion bag to contain 1 mg of drug. The patient is 66 kg. What dose is the patient receiving?

---

A diabetic patient needs to be administered insulin via continuous infusion. Pharmacy delivers an infusion bag with 250 units in 500 cc of NS. The physician orders 11 u/hr for this 90 kg patient. What rate will you run this infusion at?

Date: _____

A patient you are caring for needs to be administered an infusion of nipride at 8 mcg/kg/min. The patient weighs 80 kg. You have 50 mg of nipride available and a 250 cc IV bag. What rate will you run this infusion at?

A patient is in shock and you need to administer epinephrine. You will administer 5 mcg/min. Your plan is to mix 1 mg of 1:1000 epi into a 250 cc IV bag. The patient is 70 kg. What rate will you run this infusion at?

You are transporting a patient currently receiving dobutamine at a rate of 13 cc/hr. The 250 cc IV bag has a label that reads "250 mg of dobutamine". The patient weight is 88 kg. What dose is the patient receiving?

# SHIFT 36

Date: _____

---

A neuro patient is in your care and propofol is chosen for continued sedation. You decide to start with 16 mcg/kg/min. The bottle comes with 1000 mg in 100 cc. The patient weighs 65 kg. What rate will you run this infusion at?

---

Labetalol has been chosen for your hypertensive emergency patient. You have 1 gram available and will use a 250 cc IV bag. Your patient weighs 95 kg. You decide to begin the dose at 4 mg/min. What rate will you run this infusion at?

---

Amiodarone is infusing for a patient with SVT at 20 cc/hr. The sending facility has provided you with a 250 cc D5W containing 900 mg of amiodarone. The patient weighs 87 kg. What dose is the patient receiving?

## SHIFT 37

Date: _____

Heparin 20,000 units in 250 mL D5W is ordered to run at 1,250 units/hour. The patient is 73 kg. What rate will you run this infusion at?

A MD wants you to continue a fentanyl drip for an intubated cancer patient targeting 300 mcg/hr. Three (3) mg of fentanyl was injected into a 250 cc D5W IV bag. The patient weighs 70 kg. What rate will you run this infusion at?

You patient requires sedation while on the mechanical ventilator, and you decide to administer propofol. On hand, you have a glass bottle with 1000 mg dissolved into a 100 cc lipid emulsion. You decide to start the infusion at 12 mcg/mg/hr. The patient is 91 kg. What rate will you run this infusion at?

# SHIFT 38

Date: _____

---

A patient is receiving a lidocaine drip. The order is for 2 mg per minute. One gram of lidocaine has been added to a 500 mL IV bag. The patient weighs 85 kg. What rate will you run this infusion at?

---

You need to administer insulin to your DKA patient and decide 2 u/hr is needed. The patient weighs 68 kg. Pharmacy has prepared for you an IV bag of 500 NS with 100 units injected into it. What rate will you run this infusion at?

---

An angina patient is receiving nitroglycerin at 10 cc/hr. The pharmacy mixed the drip and you note the 250 cc D5W IV bag to have 100 mg of nitroglycerin in it. Your patient is 72 kg. What dose is the patient receiving?

## SHIFT 39

Date: _____

A hypotensive patient requires norepinephrine. On hand, you have 5 mg and 250 cc of NS. You wish to administer 7 mcg/min. The patient weighs 80 kg. What rate will you run this infusion at?

A patient with a pulmonary embolus is receiving streptokinase. The protocol states 400k IU should be injected into a 250 cc bag of NS and be delivered at 150k IU/hr. Your patient weighs 98 kg. What rate will you run this infusion at?

Your septic patient is hypotensive. You choose Levophed and decide to administer 17 mcg/min. On hand you have 12 mg of drug, a 250 cc IV bag of NS, and a patient weighing 69 kg. What rate will you run this infusion at?

# SHIFT 40

Date: _____

---

A patient requires Brevibloc for tachycardia. The order calls for 20 mcg/kg/min. On hand, you have 500 mg in 250 cc of D5W. The patient weighs 97 kg. What rate will you run this infusion at?

---

Amiodarone is infusing for a patient with SVT at 50 cc/hr. The sending facility has provided you with a 250 cc D5W containing 500 mg of amiodarone. The patient weighs 87 kg. What dose is the patient receiving?

---

Your patient with 2nd degree heart block is receiving isuprel at 75 cc/hr. The infusion bag looks to have 5 mg in 250 cc of NS. Your patient weighs 68 kg. What dose is the patient receiving?

# SHIFT 41

Date: _____

An angina patient is receiving nitroglycerin at 5 cc/hr. The pharmacy mixed the drip and you note the 500 cc D5W IV bag to have 65 mg of nitroglycerin in it. Your patient is 54 kg. What dose is the patient receiving?

Your septic patient is hypotensive. You choose Levophed and decide to administer 15 mcg/min. On hand you have 5 mg of drug, a 500 cc IV bag of NS, and a patient weighing 85 kg. What rate will you run this infusion at?

Dobutamine needs to be administered to a heart failure patient. You have a vial of 250 mg of dobutamine and a 250 cc IV bag of NS. The patient weighs 88 kg. You decide to administer 10 mcg/kg/min. What rate will you run this infusion at?

# SHIFT 42

Date: _____

---

Dobutamine needs to be administered to a heart failure patient. You have a vial of 500 mg of dobutamine and a 500 cc IV bag of NS. The patient weighs 75 kg. You decide to administer 6 mcg/kg/min. What rate will you run this infusion at?

---

A patient requires a heparin infusion and has already received the bolus. The MD is asking for 750 units/h. The pre-mixed bag is supplied with 50,000 units in 250 cc of D5W. Your patient is 70 kg. A nurse in the room suggests the correct rate to be 24 cc/hr. Is this correct?

---

A diabetic patient needs to be administered insulin via continuous infusion. Pharmacy delivers an infusion bag with 250 units in 500 cc of NS. The physician orders 11 u/hr for this 78 kg patient, and you observe the IV pump running at 9 cc/hr. Is this the correct infusion rate? If not, how would you correct it?

Date: _____

A hypotensive patient has a neosynepherine drip running at 10 cc/hr. You note the 500 cc infusion bag to contain 3 mg of drug. The patient is 85 kg. The medical staff reports the medication is infusing at 15 mcg/min. Is the patient receiving the correct dose? If not, how would you correct it??

A patient you are caring for needs to be administered an infusion of nipride at 5 mcg/kg/min. The patient weighs 75 kg. You have 25 mg of nipride available and a 250 cc IV bag. What rate will you run this infusion at? An app on your phone indicates the rate should be 50 cc/hr. Is the app correct?

A patient is in shock and you need to administer epinephrine. You will administer 5 mcg/ min. Your plan is to mix 2 mg of 1:1000 epi into a 500 cc IV bag. The patient is 103 kg. After examining some drug tables, your partner suggests a rate of 35 cc/hr. Is he correct?

# SHIFT 44

Date: _____

A patient requires a heparin infusion and has already received the bolus. The MD is asking for 1000 units/h. The pre-mixed bag is supplied with 50,000 units in 500 cc of D5W. Your patient is 95 kg. What rate will you run this infusion at?

Dopamine is being infused to a hypotensive patient at 20 cc/hr. The patient is 80 kg. Pharmacy has mixed the 250 cc NS IV bag with 750 mg. What dose is the patient receiving?

A hypotensive patient has a neosynepherine drip running at 10 cc/hr. You note the 500 cc infusion bag to contain 1 mg of drug. The patient is 88 kg. The medical staff reports the medication is infusing at 7 mcg/min. Is the patient receiving the correct dose? If not, how would you correct it?

## SHIFT 45

Date: _____

---

Amiodarone is infusing for a patient with SVT at 20 cc/hr. The sending facility has provided you with a 250 cc D5W containing 500 mg of amiodarone. The patient weighs 77 kg. What dose is the patient receiving?

---

A patient is receiving a lidocaine drip. The order is for 3 mg per minute. One gram of lidocaine has been added to a 500 mL IV bag. The patient weighs 93 kg. What rate will you run this infusion at?

---

A stroke patient is in your care and propofol is chosen for continued sedation. You decide to start with 12 mcg/kg/min. The bottle comes with 1000 mg in 100 cc. The patient weighs 88 kg. Your partner thinks the IV pump should be set to 15 cc/hr. Is your partner correct? If not, what can be done to correct it?

# SHIFT 46

Date: _____

---

Labetalol has been chosen for your hypertensive emergency patient. You have 2 gram available and will use a 250 cc IV bag. Your patient weighs 87 kg. You decide to begin the dose at 5 mg/min. What rate will you run this infusion at?

---

A hypotensive patient requires norepinephrine. On hand, you have 10 mg and 500 cc of NS. You wish to administer 25 mcg/min. The patient weighs 74 kg. What rate will you run this infusion at?

---

A patient requires a heparin infusion and has already received the bolus. The MD is asking for 1000 units/h. The pre-mixed bag is supplied with 50,000 units in 250 cc of D5W. Your patient is 93 kg. A nurse in the room suggests the correct rate to be 15 cc/hr. Is this correct? If not, how would you correct it?

## SHIFT 47

Date: _____

Norepinephrine is being run at 20 cc/hr. The IV bag reads 8 mg in 250 of normal saline. The patient weighs 77 kg. What dose is the patient receiving?

Dopamine is being infused to a hypotensive patient at 5 cc/hr. The patient is 98 kg. Pharmacy has mixed the 500 cc NS IV bag with 750 mg. What dose is the patient receiving?

You are transporting a patient currently receiving dobutamine at a rate of 30 cc/hr. The IV bag has 250 mg in 100 cc D5W. The patient weight is 88 kg. What dose is the patient receiving? The sending medical staff reports the patient is receiving 15 mcg/kg/min. Is the patient receiving the correct dose? If not, how would you correct it?

# SHIFT 48

Date: _____

---

A hypotensive patient has a neosynepherine drip running at 10 cc/hr. You note the 50 cc infusion bag to contain 1 mg of drug. The patient is 86 kg. What dose is the patient receiving?

---

You need to administer insulin to your DKA patient and decide 8 u/hr is needed. The patient weighs 100 kg. Pharmacy has prepared for you an IV bag of 250 NS with 100 units injected into it. What rate will you run this infusion at?

---

A diabetic patient needs to be administered insulin via continuous infusion. Pharmacy delivers an infusion bag with 300 units in 500 cc of NS. The physician orders 10 u/hr for this 84 kg patient, and you observe the IV pump running at 20 cc/hr. Is this the correct infusion rate? If not, how would you correct it?

## SHIFT 49

Date: _____

---

Heparin 20,000 units in 500 mL D5W is ordered to run at 1,000 units/hour. The patient is 89 kg. What rate will you run this infusion at?

---

Amiodarone is infusing for a patient with SVT at 12 cc/hr. The sending facility has provided you with a 250 cc D5W containing 1000 mg of amiodarone. The patient weighs 72 kg. What dose is the patient receiving?

---

A patient is in shock and you need to administer epinephrine. You will administer 11 mcg/ min. Your plan is to mix 1 mg of 1:1000 epi into a 250 cc IV bag. The patient is 99 kg. After examining some drug tables, your partner suggests a rate of 165 cc/hr. Is he correct?

# SHIFT 50

Date: _____

---

A diabetic patient needs to be administered insulin via continuous infusion. Pharmacy delivers an infusion bag with 300 units in 275 cc of NS. The physician orders 9 u/hr for this 85 kg patient. What rate will you run this infusion at?

---

Norepinephrine is being run at 20 cc/hr. The IV bag reads 2 mg in 500 of normal saline. The patient weighs 95 kg. What dose is the patient receiving?

---

A patient you are caring for needs to be administered an infusion of nipride at 3 mcg/kg/min. The patient weighs 95 kg. You have 100 mg of nipride available and a 500 cc IV bag. What rate will you run this infusion at? An app on your phone indicates the rate should be 85 cc/hr. Is the app correct?

Date: _____

A patient is receiving a lidocaine drip. The order is for 2 mg per minute. One gram of lidocaine has been added to a 250 mL IV bag. The patient weighs 93 kg. What rate will you run this infusion at?

Your patient with 2nd degree heart block is receiving isuprel at 75 cc/hr. The infusion bag looks to have 5 mg in 250 cc of NS. Your patient weighs 82 kg. What dose is the patient receiving?

Labetalol has been chosen for your hypertensive emergency patient. You have 1 gram available and will use a 250 cc IV bag. Your patient weighs 76 kg. You decide to begin the dose at 5 mg/min. You first calculated the needed infusion rate as 60 cc/hr, but you feel this may be high. Is your suspicion warranted, or was your original calculation correct?

# SHIFT 52

Date: _____

A patient is in shock and you need to administer epinephrine. You will administer 11 mcg/ min. Your plan is to mix 1 mg of 1:1000 epi into a 250 cc IV bag. The patient is 75 kg. What rate will you run this infusion at?

Nipride is being delivered at 50 cc/hr. The patient weighs 100 kg. On hand, you have 50 mg of Nipride in a 500 cc glass bottle of 0.9% saline. What dose is the patient receiving?

You are transporting a patient currently receiving dobutamine at a rate of 17 cc/hr. The IV bag which was mixed by their pharmacy has 358 mg in 50 of D5W. The patient weight is 95 kg. What dose is the patient receiving? The sending medical staff reports the patient is receiving 16 mcg/kg/min. Is the patient receiving the correct dose? If not, how would you correct it?

## SHIFT 53

Date: _____

A MD wants you to continue a fentanyl drip for an intubated cancer patient targeting 400 mcg/hr. Four (4) mg of fentanyl was injected into a 250 cc D5W IV bag. The patient weighs 69 kg. What rate will you run this infusion at?

A patient requires Brevibloc for tachycardia. The order calls for 35 mcg/kg/min. On hand, you have 1250 mg in 250 cc of D5W. The patient weighs 99 kg. What rate will you run this infusion at?

Your patient is receiving a continuous infusion of neosynepherine at 17 cc/hr. The patient is 80 kg. You have injected 20 mg into a 250 cc NS IV bag. It is reported that the patient is receiving a dose of 10 mcg/min. Is this correct? If not, how would you correct it??

## SHIFT 54

Date: _____

A patient you are caring for needs to be administered an infusion of Nipride at 10 mcg/kg/min. The patient weighs 93 kg. You have 50 mg of Nipride available and a 500 cc IV bag. What rate will you run this infusion at?

A patient with a pulmonary embolus is receiving streptokinase. The protocol states 700k IU should be injected into a 250 cc bag of NS and be delivered at 100k IU/hr. Your patient weighs 98 kg. What rate will you run this infusion at?

A patient requires a heparin infusion and has already received the bolus. The MD is asking for 400 units/h. The pre-mixed bag is supplied with 50,000 units in 500 cc of D5W. Your patient is 78 kg. A nurse in the room suggests the correct rate to be 15 cc/hr. Is this correct? If not, how would you correct it?

Date: _____

The IV pump reads "17 cc/hr". Your patient is receiving a continuous infusion of neosynepherine. You have injected 12 mg into a 250 cc NS IV bag. The patient is 75 kg. What dose is the patient receiving?

An angina patient is receiving nitroglycerin at 11 cc/hr. The pharmacy mixed the drip and you note the 500 cc D5W IV bag to have 100 mg of nitroglycerin in it. Your patient is 78 kg. What dose is the patient receiving?

A stroke patient is in your care and propofol is chosen for continued sedation. You decide to start with 27 mcg/kg/min. The bottle comes with 1000 mg in 100 cc. The patient weighs 65 kg. Your partner thinks the IV pump should be set to 25 cc/hr. Is your partner correct? If not, what can be done to correct it?

# SHIFT 56

Date: _____

---

Your septic patient is hypotensive. You choose Levophed and decide to administer 18 mcg/min. On hand you have 8 mg of drug, a 250 cc IV bag of NS, and a patient weighing 87 kg. What rate will you run this infusion at?

---

You are transporting a patient currently receiving dobutamine at a rate of 21 cc/hr. The 250 cc IV bag has a label that reads "600 mg of dobutamine". The patient weight is 74 kg. What dose is the patient receiving?

---

A diabetic patient needs to be administered insulin via continuous infusion. Pharmacy delivers an infusion bag with 100 units in 250 cc of NS. The physician orders 10 u/hr for this 70 kg patient, and you observe the IV pump running at 17 cc/hr. Is this the correct infusion rate? If not, how would you correct it?

## SHIFT 57

Date: _____

A patient is receiving a lidocaine drip. The order is for 3 mg per minute. One gram of lidocaine has been added to a 250 mL IV bag. The patient weighs 71 kg. What rate will you run this infusion at?

A neuro patient is in your care and propofol is chosen for continued sedation. You decide to start with 10 mcg/kg/min. The bottle comes with 1000 mg in 100 cc. The patient weighs 89 kg. What rate will you run this infusion at?

A patient is in shock and you need to administer epinephrine. You will administer 15 mcg/min. Your plan is to mix 1 mg of 1:1000 epi into a 500 cc IV bag. The patient is 85 kg. After examining some drug tables, your partner suggests a rate of 20 cc/hr. Is he correct?

# SHIFT 58

Date: _____

A hypotensive patient requires norepinephrine. On hand, you have 7 mg and 500 cc of NS. You wish to administer 15 mcg/min. The patient weighs 88 kg. What rate will you run this infusion at?

You patient requires sedation while on the mechanical ventilator, and you decide to administer propofol. On hand, you have a glass bottle with 1000 mg dissolved into a 100 cc lipid emulsion. You decide to start the infusion at 24 mcg/mg/hr. The patient is 76 kg. What rate will you run this infusion at?

A patient you are caring for needs to be administered an infusion of Nipride at 1 mcg/kg/min. The patient weighs 79 kg. You have 50 mg of Nipride available and a 250 cc IV bag. What rate will you run this infusion at? An app on your phone indicates the rate should be 45 cc/hr. Is the app correct?

## SHIFT 59

Date: _____

Your patient requires sedation while on the mechanical ventilator, and you decide to administer propofol. On hand, you have a glass bottle with 1000 mg dissolved into a 100 cc lipid emulsion. You decide to start the infusion at 30 mcg/mg/hr. The patient is 70 kg. What rate will you run this infusion at?

Doubutamine needs to be administered to a heart failure patient. You have a vial of 250 mg of dobutamine and a 500 cc IV bag of NS. The patient weighs 85 kg. You decide to administer 11 mcg/kg/min. What rate will you run this infusion at?

Labetalol has been chosen for your hypertensive emergency patient. You have 2 gram available and will use a 250 cc IV bag. Your patient weighs 88 kg. You decide to begin the dose at 2 mg/min. You first calculated the needed infusion rate as 46 cc/hr, but you feel this may be high. Is your suspicion warranted, or was your original calculation correct?

# SHIFT 60

Date: _____

---

A patient with a pulmonary embolus is receiving streptokinase. The protocol states 550k IU should be injected into a 250 cc bag of NS and be delivered at 75k IU/hr. Your patient weighs 99 kg. What rate will you run this infusion at?

---

An angina patient is receiving nitroglycerin at 10 cc/hr. The pharmacy mixed the drip and you note the 250 cc D5W IV bag to have 100 mg of nitroglycerin in it. Your patient is 89 kg. What dose is the patient receiving?

---

Your patient is 77 kg. You have injected 15 mg into a 250 cc NS IV bag. It is reported that the patient is receiving a dose of 20 mcg/min. Is this correct? If not, how would you correct it?

# 9 SHIFT PRACTICE ANSWERS

Shift 1:
1. 8 cc/hr
2. 0.2 mcg/min
3. 8.25 cc/hr

Shift 2:
1. 152 cc/hr
2. 90 cc/hr
3. 1.6 mcg/kg/min

Shift 3:
1. 3.4 cc/hr
2. 60 cc/hr
3. 0.5 mg/min

Shift 4:
1. 27 cc/hr
2. 27 cc/hr
3. 5.8 cc/hr

Shift 5:
1. 30 cc/hr
2. 11.8 cc/hr
3. 20.8 cc/hr

Shift 6:
1. 56.3 cc/hr
2. 62.5 cc/hr
3. 45 cc/hr

Shift 7:
1. 58.3 cc/hr
2. 0.7 mg/min
3. 20 mcg/min

Shift 8:
1. 11.6 cc/hr
2. 20.6 cc/hr
3. 20.4 cc/hr

Shift 9:
1. 9.8 cc/hr
2. Not correct. 8 cc/hr gets 800 u/hr, so 15 cc/hr is about double. To correct, set IV pump to 8 cc/hr.
3. The IV pump is running too slow (at 5.5 cc/hr). Doubling the rate to 11 cc/hr gets you very close to delivering 7 u/hr. To exactly deliver 7 u/hr, you'd need to set the pump at 11.5 cc/hr).

Shift 10:
1. At 5cc/hr the patient is only receiving 0.16 mcg/min. In this case, simply work the problem from the forwards direction. 300 cc/hr at the provided concentration would achieve 10 mcg/min.
2. The app is not correct. The correct rate is 108 cc/hr. Doubling the app's suggestion would arrive much closer to the correct rate.
3. Your partner is not correct. The correct rate would be 49.5 cc/hr to deliver the dose of 6 mcg/min at the provided concentration. To correct if your partner set up the IV pump at 16.3, you could triple this rate to 49 cc/hr. At 16.3

cc/hr, you are only delivering 1.98 mcg/min.

Shift 11:
1. 8 cc/hr
2. 6.7 cc/hr
3. The patient is actually receiving 0.53 mcg/min at 8 cc/hr. So, to get the dose to the desired 10 mcg/min, you'd have to multiply 20 to the rate (because 20 x 0.5 mcg/min is 10 mcg/min). So, 20 x 8 cc/hr = 160 cc/hr would deliver about 10 mcg/min from this quick fix. The math exactly works out to 150 cc/hr delivers 10 mcg/min, and 160 cc/hr delivers 10.6 mcg/min. Either way (150 or 160 cc/hr) you are within the ballpark.

Shift 12:
1. 0.75 mg/min
2. 75 cc/hr
3. Your partner is wrong again. A rate of 10 cc/hr would deliver a dose of 22.2 mcg/kg/min. To deliver 9 mcg/kg/min, you'd need to set the pump to 4.1 cc/hr.

Shift 13:
1. 120 cc/hr
2. 57.9 cc/hr
3. The RN is wrong and is off by a factor of about

3. The correct rate is 3.75 cc/hr to deliver 750 u/hr at the provided concentration.

Shift 14:
1. 1.8 mcg/min
2. 9.9 mcg/kg/min
3. The patient is receiving 11.8 cc/hr, so yes. They are receiving the correct dose.

Shift 15:
1. 0.17 mg/min
2. 1.7 cc/hr
3. The patient is actually receiving 5.4 u/hr at a rate of 9 cc/hr. So if we half both we'd get 2.7 u/hr at a rate of 4.5 cc/hr. add 2.7 u/hr to the original dose of 5.4 u/hr to obtain 8.1 u/hr. So the same for the rate, add 9 cc/hr to 4.5 cc/hr to yield 13.5 cc/hr. Therefore, changing the rate to 13.5 cc/hr would achieve a dosing of 8 u/hr with the provided concentration.

Shift 16:
1. 37.5 cc/hr
2. 0.6 mg/min
3. Your partner is very wrong in this case. The IV pump needs to be set at 135 cc/hr to be delivering 9 mcg/min at the provided concentration.

Shift 17:
1. 8.25 cc/hr
2. 2.6 mcg/min
3. The app is very close, 57 cc/hr delivers 2 mcg/kg/min. it'd be safe to start at this rate.

Shift 18:
1. 90 cc/hr
2. 20 mcg/min
3. Your original calculation is correct. The correct rate for a dosing of 4 mg/min at the provided concentration.

Shift 19:
1. 210 cc/hr
2. 1.9 mcg/kg/min
3. The patient is actually receiving 5.5 mcg/kg/min, so you need to double this. By doubling the rate, you'll double this dose to 11 mcg/kg/min, which is pretty close to 12 mcg/kg/min. Or you could just work out the problem forwardly and obtain 45.9 cc/hr will deliver 12 mcg/kg/min.

Shift 20:
1. 8.3 cc/hr
2. 41.6 cc/hr
3. This is perfect. The patient is receiving the desired dose of 13 mcg/min.

Shift 21:
1. 528 cc/hr
2. 45 cc/hr
3. The patient should actually receive 2.5 cc.hr to achieve 500 units/hr with 50,000 units in a 250 cc IV bag. You could politely correct the staff that its 2.5 cc/hr, or just say thanks and silently make the change. That's what I routinely do.

Shift 22:
1. 15.3 mcg/min
2. 53.3 mcg/min
3. No, the correct rate to deliver 11 mcg/kg/min is 5.8 cc/hr. If 20 cc/hr were on the pump and infusing, then you'd need to change it to 5.8 cc/hr.

Shift 23:
1. 31.5 cc/hr
2. 10.8 mcg/kg/min
3. No, the rate is incorrect. The correct rate is 10 u/hr.

Shift 24:
1. 60 cc/hr
2. 2.6 cc/hr
3. No, the correct rate 300 cc/hr to achieve the desired dose.

Shift 25:
1. 48 cc/hr
2. 8.1 cc/hr

3. No, the app is wrong. The correct infusion rate is 237 cc/hr.

Shift 26:
1. 15.2 cc/hr
2. 112.2 cc/hr
3. You are very close. A dose of 2 mg/min with the concentration provided will yield an infusion rate of 60 cc/min. To achieve the desired dose, simply increase your flow rate from 55 cc/hr to 60 cc/hr.

Shift 27:
1. 45 cc/hr
2. 66.6 mcg/min
3. The actual dose the patient is receiving is 30 mcg/min. So, no, they are not receiving 15 mcg/min, they are receiving twice that. To correct this reduce the infusion rate by half (change to 11.5 cc/hr).

Shift 28:
1. 12.5 cc/hr
2. 20.83 mcg/min
3. Close. The IV pump should be set to 14.4 cc/hr.

Shift 29:
1. 46.66 cc/hr
2. 15 cc/hr
3. No. That patient is actually receiving 15.4

mcg/kg/min. To deliver 10 mcg/kg/min, you'd need to dial in 35.7 cc/hr.

Shift 30:
1. 64.5 cc/hr
2. 105.6 cc/hr
3. Actually, this is too slow of a rate. To deliver the 3 mg/min with the provided concentration, you would need to set the pump rate to 90 cc/hr.

Shift 31:
1. 5.2 cc/hr
2. 0.53 mcg/min
3. 11 cc/hr

Shift 32:
1. 152.1 cc/hr
2. 90 cc/hr
3. 1.65 mcg/kg/min

Shift 33:
1. 4 cc/hr
2. 0.2 mcg/min
3. No. The drug tables are way off. You'd need to set the IV pump at a rate of 135 cc/hr to deliver 9mcg/min.

Shift 34:
1. 3.5 cc/hr
2. 0.166 mcg/min
3. 22 cc/hr

Shift 35:
1. 192 cc/hr
2. 75 cc/hr

3.  2.5 mcg/kg/min

Shift 36:
1.  6.24 cc/hr
2.  60 cc/hr
3.  1.2 mg/min

Shift 37:
1.  15.6 cc/hr
2.  25 cc/hr
3.  6.55 cc/hr

Shift 38:
1.  60 cc/hr
2.  2 cc/hr
3.  66.6 mcg/min

Shift 39:
1.  21 cc/hr
2.  93.75 cc/hr
3.  21.25 cc/hr

Shift 40:
1.  58.2 cc/hr
2.  1.66 mg/min
3.  25 mcg/min, or 0.37 mcg/kg/min. The first doesn't account for the patient's weight and the second does.

Shift 41:
1.  10.8 mcg/min
2.  30 cc/hr
3.  1.89 mcg/kg/min

Shift 42:
1.  1.33 cc/hr
2.  No. She would be administering 8 times the order. The correct rate for the IV pump would be 3.75 cc/hr.
3.  This is NOT the correct infusion rate. A rate of 9 cc/hr would deliver 4.5 u/hr. The correct rate with this concentration would be 22 cc/hr to deliver the ordered 11 u/hr.

Shift 43:
1.  No. The patient is actually receiving 1 mcg/min. At this concentration, a rate of 150 cc/hr would be needed to administer 15 mcg/min.
2.  225 cc/hr is the rate needed to achieve 5 mcg/kg/min. The app is wrong or a number was mis-typed.
3.  No. The actual rate needed is 75 cc/hr. You'd be close if you doubled their suggestion.

Shift 44:
1.  100 cc/hr
2.  12.5 cc/hr
3.  0.33 cc/hr

Shift 45:
1.  0.66 mg/min
2.  90 cc/hr
3.  No, your partner is wrong. The correct rate would be 6.34 cc/hr. His dose is over double the dose.

Shift 46:
1. 37.5 cc/hr
2. 75 cc/hr
3. No, 15 cc/hr is NOT correct. The correct rate would be 5 cc/hr.

Shift 47:
1. 10.66 mcg/min
2. 1.28 mcg/kg/min
3. Very close. The patient is actually receiving 14.2 mcg/kg/min. You could change the rate to 31.7 cc/hr to for sure give 15 mcg/kg/min, or just see if the slightly lower dose is therapeutic.

Shift 48:
1. 3.3 mcg/min
2. 20 cc/hr
3. No. The correct infusion rate is 16.67. Change the pump rate to 16.67.

Shift 49:
1. 25 cc/hr.
2. 0.8 mcg/min
3. Yes, he is correct. The rate is 165 cc/hr.

Shift 50:
1. 8.25 cc/hr
2. 1.33 mcg/min
3. Yes the app is correct. 85.5 cc/hr is the correct rate.

Shift 51:
1. 30 cc/hr
2. 0.3 mcg/kg/min
3. Your suspicion is warranted, but your first calculation is too low. The rate of 60 cc/hr would be too low. The rate needed is 75 cc/hr. this would deliver the ordered 5mg/min.

Shift 52:
1. 165 cc/hr
2. 0.83 mcg/kg/min
3. The patient is receiving 21.4 mcg/kg/min. The staff is wrong, but not by much. If the patient is to receive 16 mcg/kg/min with this weird concentration/mix, then the rate would need to be 12.7 cc/hr.

Shift 53:
1. 25 cc/hr
2. 41.58 cc/hr
3. 22.67 mcg/min

Shift 54:
1. 558 cc/hr, which isn't an ideal rate because of so much fluid.
2. 35.7 cc/hr
3. The nurse is wrong. The correct rate is 4 cc/hr.

Shift 55:
1. 13.6 mcg/min
2. 36.66 mcg/min
3. Your partner is wrong. The correct rate is 10.53 cc/hr.

Shift 56:
1. 33.75 cc/hr

2. 11.35 mcg/kg/min
3. No. The correct rate would be 25 cc/hr.

Shift 57:
1. 45 cc/hr
2. 5.34 cc/hr
3. No. The correct rate with the given concentration is 450 cc/hr.

Shift 58:
1. 64.28 cc/hr
2. 10.94 cc/hr
3. No. The correct rate is 23.7 cc/hr to deliver 1 mcg/kg/min.

Shift 59:
1. 12.6 cc/hr
2. 112.2 cc/hr
3. Your suspicion is warranted. The correct rate is 15 cc/hr.

Shift 60:
1. 34 cc/hr
2. 66.66 mcg/min
3. This is correct. This is an interesting case where the rate and dose are the same, but the concentration isn't mixed 1:1. Here, 20 cc/hr will deliver 20 mcg/min.

# ABOUT THE AUTHOR

Charlie Swearingen first conceived the dream of becoming a flight clinician while he was still in paramedic school. He decided that instead of blithely waiting for a position to become available, he would begin arming himself with the professional achievements that would eventually earn him a spot on a revered, level 1 helicopter in Mississippi. He is in the middle of a PhD in physiology, is an educator for the world's largest air medical service provider, and also is a world class athlete on the US National Men's Sitting volleyball team. He eventually founded Meducation Specialists, a company dedicated to developing and deploying world-class medical education.

Made in the USA
Columbia, SC
12 April 2025

56512949R00087